Disclaimer

This book is informational only. The information is not intended for use in connection with the sale of any product. Any claims or presentations regarding any specific products or brand names are strictly the responsibility of the product owners or manufacturers. This summary of information from unpublished sources, books, research journals and articles is not intended to replace the advice or attention of health care professionals. It is not intended to direct their behavior or replace their independent professional judgment. If you have a problem with your health, or before you embark on any health, fitness or sports training programs, seek clearance from a qualified health care professional.

Cover Model: *Gary Strydom is a South African/Afrikaner and an accomplished IFBB professional bodybuilder whose career spans three decades. At 54 years old, Gary made a comeback in 2006, setting the world abuzz with his dynamic new look proving that the sport of bodybuilding is "ageless." Read more about Gary's amazing bodybuilding career at:*

http://garystrydom.com/index.php/about-gary-strydom/

Table of Contents

Chapter I: History

Brief History

It would be nice to say this is the first book written on dumbbell training, but we were beaten to the punch by nearly 1800 years!

In 200 A.D., Galen, a Greek physician, wrote a text detailing the virtues of dumbbell training and the potential healing power of training with dumbbells. The book was called *De Sanitate Tuenda*. *De Sanitate Tuenda* served as the proverbial "dumbbell Bible" for the next 1,500 years!

Over the last few decades, free weight training has gained acceptance among medical professionals and the masses as a way for women to improve their health and aesthetics. Roman women gained these benefits nearly two millenniums ago. Recently, a mosaic dating back to the second century A.D. was discovered depicting a Roman woman training with a somewhat contemporary-looking dumbbell.

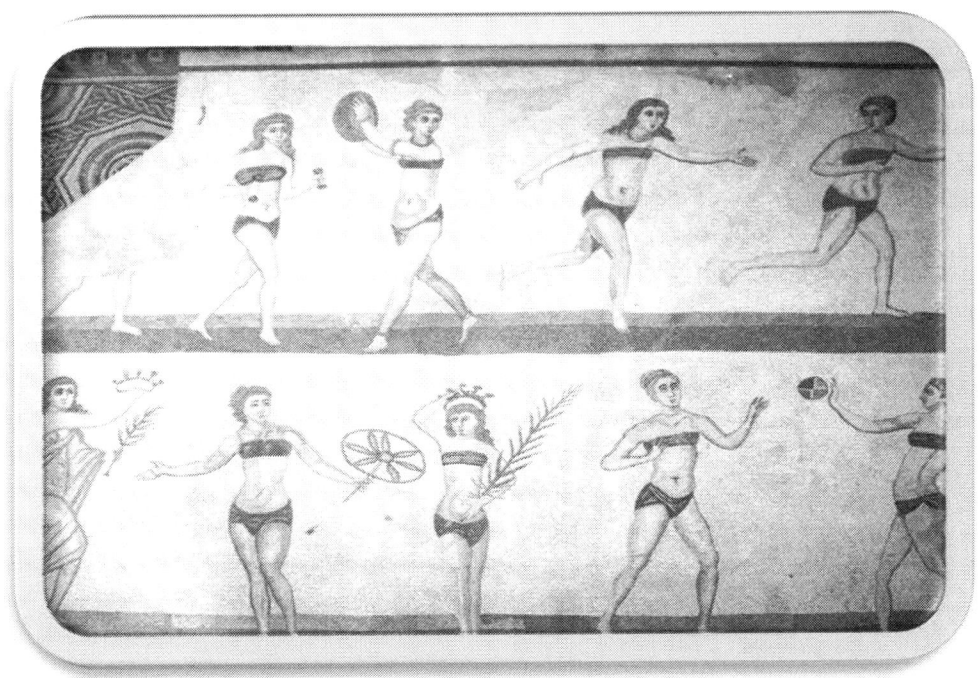

In 1569, physician Hieronymus Mercurialis wrote *De Arte Gymnastica Aput Ancientes*, a compilation of theories on medicine and exercise. Mercurialis advocated exercising with halteres (dumbbells) and heavy sand-filled bags.

Name Origin

The word "dumbbell" originated in England in the late 1600s, during the Stuart Period. Initially, this referred to a piece of equipment simulating the action of a bell rope for developing technique and especially strength for the purpose of practicing English bell ringing, but without making a noise (hence dumb). As strongmen started to make their own equipment, they kept the name, even though the shape and form changed.

On the other side of the pond, the great Benjamin Franklin, in letters to his son, wrote that, "I live temperately, drink no wine, and use daily the exercise of the dumb-bell." Thomas Jefferson trained with dumbbells to strengthen an injured wrist and quite possibly to deal with the stress of 9,999 missed attempts in developing the light bulb.

Oldie But Goodie

For thousands of years, dumbbell training has benefited general health and helped construct the strongest and most muscular physiques of all-time. In the words of Strength Sensei Charles Poliquin, "Everything old is new again, but sometimes those old things are still the best!"

We both wholeheartedly thank you for letting us be a part of your training journey. You will now have one more weapon in your arsenal with *The Complete Guide to Dumbbell Training: A Scientific Approach.*

Frederick C. Hatfield, Ph.D.
Josh Bryant, MS

Chapter II: Intro to Dumbbell Training

You may think that everyone in the gym knows how to use dumbbells. The word itself seems to imply that even a "dumbbell" knows how to use them. And for the most part, that's true. However, after both growing up in the weight room, we've grown to know dumbbell training from a more eclectic vantage point.

Consider first that there are several different kinds of dumbbells, each having unique features. There are also literally hundreds of dumbbell exercises for practically every muscle in the body and joint or multi-joint movements in all planes. Some kick ass and some are asinine!

It is impossible to discuss all of the various dumbbell training methods and exercises in a single book, so we'll stick to the most valuable and effective ones, plus a few unique ones we've learned from decades of experience in the trenches. Some of them will surprise you.

Explicit instructions, principles and philosophies are covered in this book. Our objective is to give you tools to design your own routines, but if you prefer to follow our listed routines, we have also included plenty of innovative, detailed programs.

Dumbbell Superiority

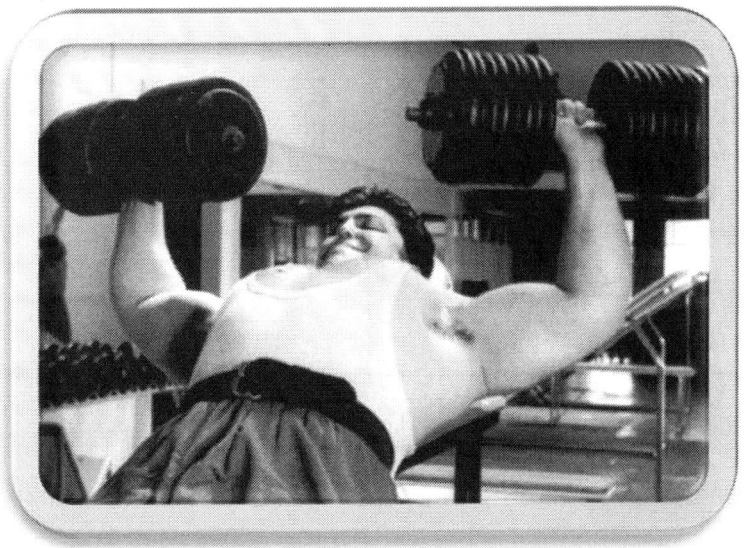

Pat Casey incline pressing 220-pound dumbbells

Contrary to the hogwash spewed at the local Curves or by the dwindling Arthur Jones nautilus "theocracy," dumbbell training is the ultimate form of weight training! There is a plethora of reasons why we believe this, and they're detailed in this book. Dumbbells reign superior to machines for many of the same reasons that barbells do.

The primary advantage dumbbells hold over machines are they allow synergistic (helping) and stabilizer muscles to come into play much more effectively than does machine training. Taking things a step further, this is also the major advantage that dumbbells have over barbells. Simply, stabilizers must act in all directions with dumbbells, whereas the barbell connects your two hands together, thereby offering a measure of greater stability.

Science Agrees

In one study, muscle activity in the free weight barbell bench press, Smith machine bench press and dumbbell bench press were measured and contrasted. The study was conducted on 12 healthy, resistance-trained young men. Researchers recorded one-repetition max and electromyographic (EMG) activity of the pectoralis major, deltoid anterior, biceps, and triceps brachii during the movements. EMG activity in the pectoralis major and anterior deltoid was similar during all three lifts. But as stability requirements increased, electrical activity in the biceps increased.

In other words, the Smith machine had the lowest activation of the biceps and the dumbbell bench press had the highest activation of the biceps because of stabilizing the load.

The study concluded that high-stability requirements in the dumbbell bench press resulted in similar EMG levels in the pectoralis major and anterior deltoids and higher biceps activation.

Saeterbakken, A. H., Van Den Tillaar, R., & Fimland, M. S. (2011). A comparison of muscle activity and 1-RM strength of three chest-press exercises with different stability requirements. Journal of Sports Sciences, 29(5), 533-538.

Science and anecdotes both agree; dumbbells have the greatest stability requirements.

Chapter III: Design Variation

Variations in Dumbbell Design

Let's identify some of the types of dumbbells that have found their way to market and then list a few unique exercises that have been done since the days when dumbbells were reintroduced into the modern era of fitness training.

Kettlebells

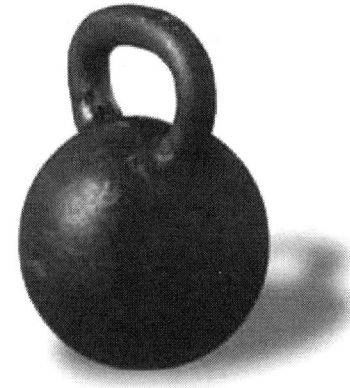

In the last decade, kettlebell training has amassed a following of biblical proportions. Many die-hard kettlebell zealots believe training with kettlebells is superior to free-weight training. To the surprise of many, some mainstream professional and college strength coaches have embraced the kettlebell. Some seem to be drinking the Kettlebell Kool Aid; others have logical arguments worth examination.

Kettlebells look sort of like a shot put or cannon ball with a handle welded to it. For hundreds of years, they have been used for strength training in Eastern Europe. If you are not sure what a kettlebell is, think of old-time cartoons like Bugs Bunny, where strongmen tossed around those odd-shaped cannon balls with handles. In the days of yesteryear, circus strongmen used these implements as part of their acts. Today, many elite athletes and overweight soccer moms are integrating kettlebell training into their strength and conditioning regimens.

Some basic exercises like the "swing" certainly can be effective for a general populace. The key to success with kettlebells training is evaluating the learning curve, the risk-to-benefit ratio and the desired training effect.

Solid Dumbbells

These were common in hotel fitness centers, until the lawyers got involved. They come with

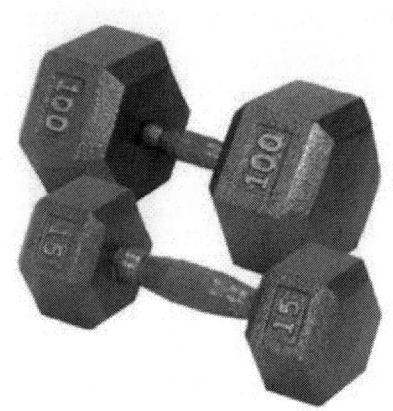

spherical ends, cylindrical ends or, more recently, octagonal ends. The octagonal dumbbells do not roll away when placed on the gym floor. While some lifters prefer the cylinders because they are more compact, there appears to be little difference in the "feel" or ease of management among the different shapes. So take your

pick!

The main advantage of solids is the fact that they are practically indestructible. More recently, the ends have been covered with rubber to prevent rusting and increase safety. An unfortunate byproduct is the lamentable loss of the clanging sound of the iron. Sort of like the loss of the much-beloved "thwack" sound when hitting a baseball with an aluminum bat.

Fixed Plate Dumbbells

Until recently, these bad boys had the market monopolized.

Think of dumbbells you started with at the YMCA, or hell, even behind bars. These dumbbells are the same as solids, except that the weights are comprised of regular exercise plates ranging from 10 pounds down to 1.25 pounds. They used to have sleeves to fit over the handle, but nowadays the handle is made anywhere from 1.25 inches in diameter to 3 inches in diameter (see

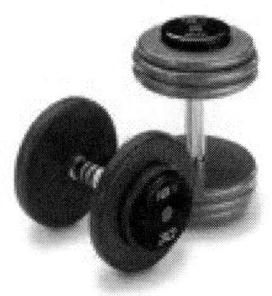

oversized grip dumbbells below). The plates are retained on the ends of the bar with screws.

The single disadvantage of this type of dumbbell is that the set screws almost always become loose or stripped when the dumbbells are dropped frequently. Keep these tightened up and enjoy the sound of those "bells" ringing!

Oversized Grip Dumbbells

Alan Calvert, one of the important forefathers of modern weight training, recommended thick handles in his 1924 book, *Super-Strength.* So they've been around awhile. In the last 20 years, with his book, *Dinosaur Training: Lost Secrets of Strength and Development*, Brooks Kubik helped ignite a resurgence in thick-handled training by talking about the benefits of using dumbbells with 2-3-inch diameter handles.

Kubik believes that the large diameter handles are better for improving gripping strength (forearm muscles as well as muscles intrinsic to the hand), an important factor in many sports.

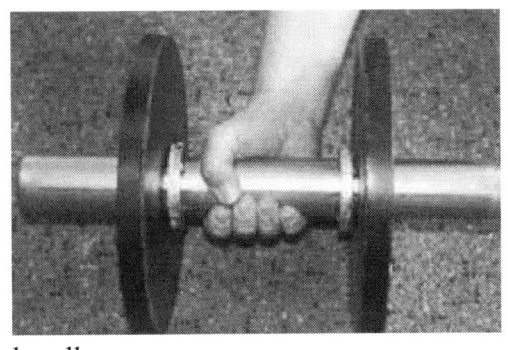

Not to mention, big forearms radiate a persona of power! Furthermore, Kubik believes that in the muscles targeted with the dumbbell exercises, more motor units (groups of muscle fibers) are activated by using the thicker handles in comparison to standard 1.25-inch handles.

Science Questions Fat Handles

A landmark 2008 study entitled, "The influence of bar diameter on neuromuscular strength and activation: Inferences from an isometric unilateral bench press" concluded: "Our data does not support the hypothesis that bar diameter influences performance during an isometric bench press exercise. Our data does not support the use of a fat bar for increasing neuromuscular activation." This has caused some to totally dismiss fat dumbbell/barbell training. Take everything with a grain of salt; this study used just a bench press, an isometric contraction (static) with a barbell. Clearly, further investigation is warranted.

Science Affirms Fat Handles

Admittedly, fat handle barbell and dumbbell training is scarce. That's how we ended up stumbling across a 1992 study published in *The International Journal of Industrial Ergonomics*. Not directed at weightlifters, this study provided invaluable insight to strength training enthusiasts by exploring the neuromuscular activity of three different diameter handles. Researchers examined the size of an industrial handle and how it affected muscular strength and neural drive, contrasting a handle matched to the inside grip diameter, a handle 1 cm smaller than the inside grip, and a handle 1 centimeter larger than the inside grip and tested electromyographic (EMG) activity (electrical activity of muscles).

Researchers learned the smallest handle required the greatest amount of voluntary muscular contraction but the lowest neuromuscular activation as assessed by EMG, in comparison to the thickest diameter handle, which triggered the greatest neuromuscular response but the smallest maximal voluntary contraction than the other two sizes.

In a nutshell, this is exactly what Kubik believed would happen. At this point, additional research is very scarce.

Fat Gripz

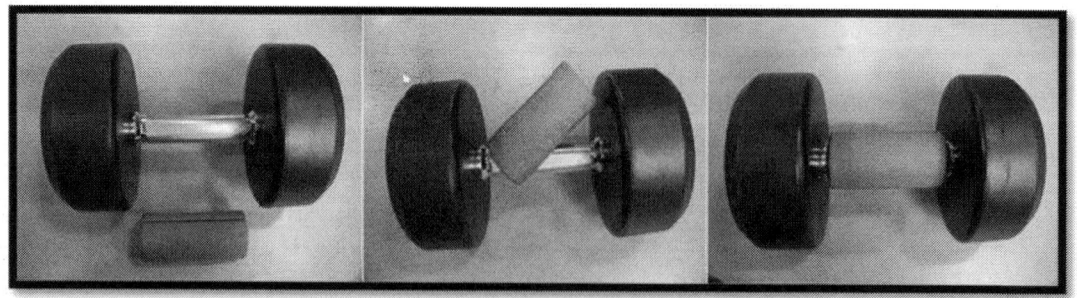

Setting up Fat Gripz on dumbbells

In the last decade, Fat Gripz have been used by thousands of athletes and military around the world for weight lifting, strength training and powerlifting, including members of the U.S. Special Forces, teams in the NFL, top MMA fighters and other elite-level athletes.

Fat Gripz are a unique training device that wraps around standard barbells, dumbbells and cable attachments, instantly and easily converting them into thick bars. Fat Gripz are made from a proprietary compound that makes them feel secure on the bar. They are designed to have no "give" or slippage whatsoever and to maintain the thick bar shape at all times so one can perform heavy compound movements.

With the exception of those training for a contest that uses a specific thick-handled barbell or dumbbell, almost any elite athlete can use Fat Gripz. They're are small, light and fully portable so they can be taken anywhere; you could carry them in your pockets onto a plane. Costing less $40, they are much more cost effective than purchasing thick-handled dumbbells.

More Benefits

Training with fat handle dumbbells, or Fat Gripz, works the weakest link (grip and forearm strength) that's holding many folks back. In theory, this modality could decrease the risk of injury because the weight's spread more evenly, putting less pressure on individual joints like the wrists and elbows. It may also minimize existing joint pain. Some top-level strength coaches anecdotally support expedited muscle hypertrophy for the entire upper body while training with Fat Gripz.

Fat-handle training offers a host of benefits, but remember, do not let targeted muscles become robbed of intended work because of added grip difficulty. Do not sacrifice rowing and shrugging poundages in the name of fat-handle work. If the goal is grip development, both of these exercises with fat handles are a great choice. If the objective is to work the upper back and traps, don't let grip be the Achilles heel; yes, even straps would be okay.

Olympic Dumbbells

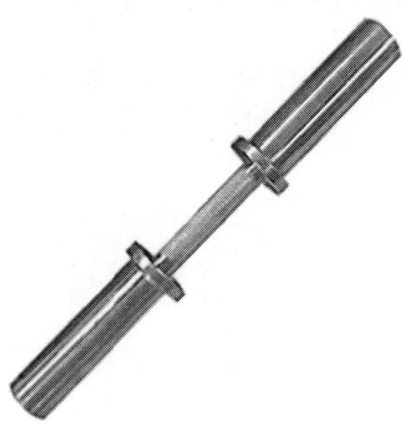

The bearing-equipped, rotating ends of an Olympic dumbbell bar offer the distinct advantage of being far more easily managed when the lifter is pulling the dumbbell(s) to the shoulders or overhead. This is because they eliminate the inertia of the moving ends of solid dumbbells. If you are performing compound (multi-joint) movements, this feature is valuable for maximizing the amount of weight you can handle.

But be careful! Make sure the collars are tight before every set.

Adjustable (Home Use) Dumbbells

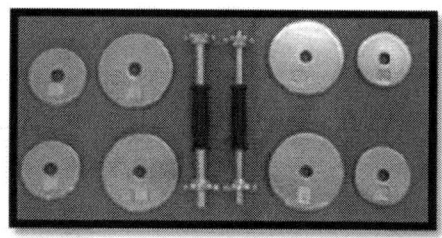

Of course, the main advantage of adjustable dumbbells is their extremely low cost in comparison to a set of fixed-weight dumbbells, and they take up little space. But be careful! Make sure the collars are tight before every set.

Iron Mind now manufactures "Big Boy Dumbbell Handles" that can hold 300-plus pounds on each dumbbell, similar to the ones legends like Pat Casey (the first man to bench press 600 pounds) and "The Mighty Minister" Paul Anderson used. Regardless of strength levels, dumbbells are non-discriminatory.

Dumbbell Stabilizer/Extender

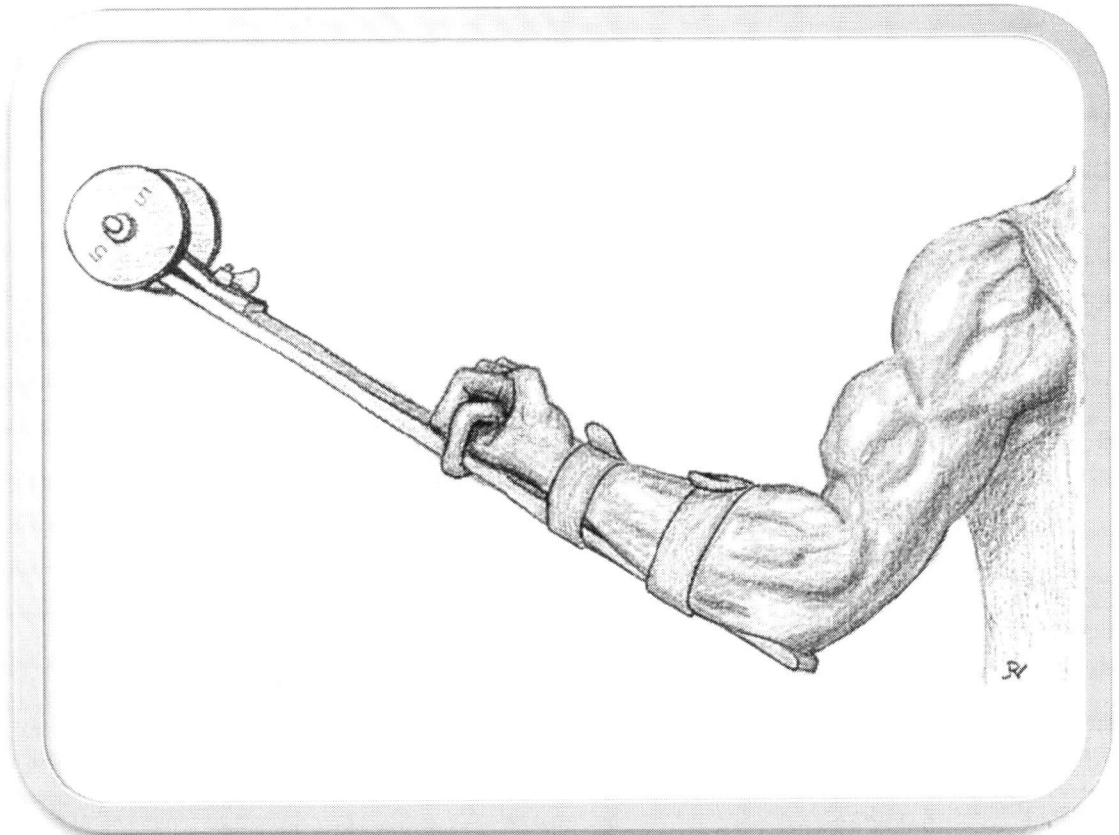

Here's another invention that hit the market somewhat recently. It consists of a built-in forearm

sleeve attachment on the dumbbell handles. Slip your hands into the sleeve and grasp the handle.

The sleeve has a cross bar that places the weight on your forearms instead of in your hands. The

device has one advantage that makes it worth mentioning. If you have arthritis or other hand or

wrist problems that make dumbbell training difficult or impossible, you can still do your

dumbbell work. Because of the increased lever arm and poor positional strength, less weight can

be used to get a similar training effect.

Rackbells

Rackbells, invented by Anthony Valentino (Rackbell Systems, Inc.) in 1996, are a refreshing improvement over regular, fixed dumbbells on at least three counts.

First, there is a built-in curved rod that spans the handle so that it is far safer and easier to spot the user. Second, the dumbbell set comes with a unique rack overhanging the user so he or she can begin by taking the dumbbells off the rack and replacing them at the end of the set in a fashion quite similar to what is done with a barbell. This is significant because lying down and getting back up with a heavy set of dumbbells is a chore none relishes, particularly novices to the iron game. It's downright scary to novices and perceived to be a task fraught with danger. The third advantage is that the dumbbells are rarely dropped, keeping them (and the floor) from being damaged.

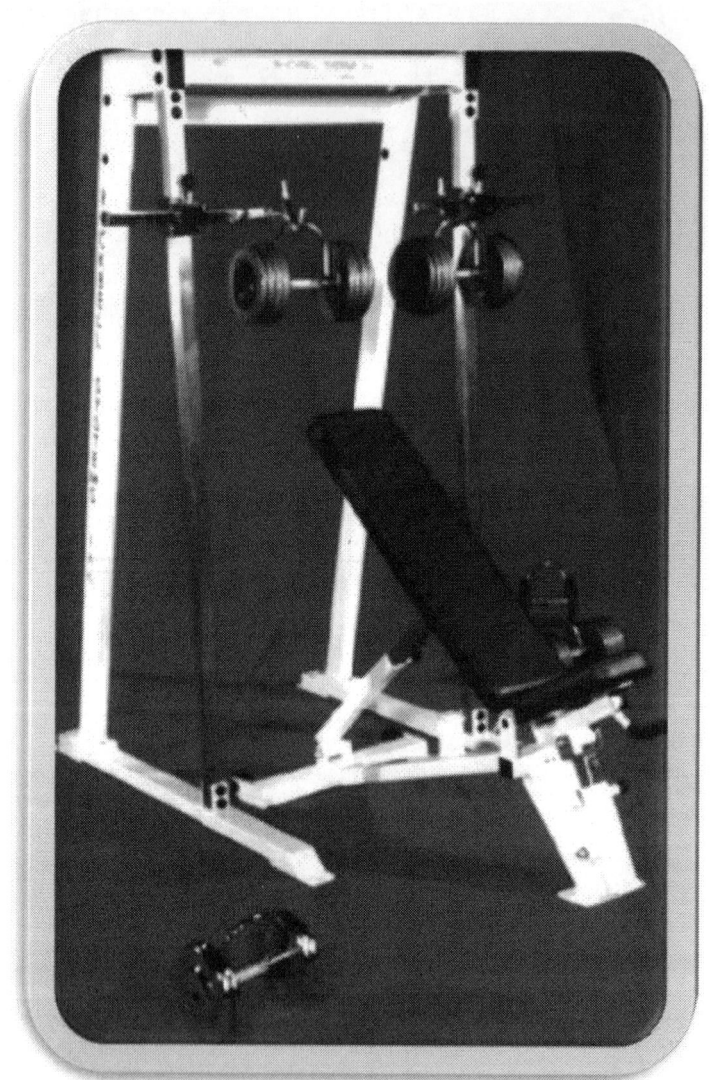

Power Hooks

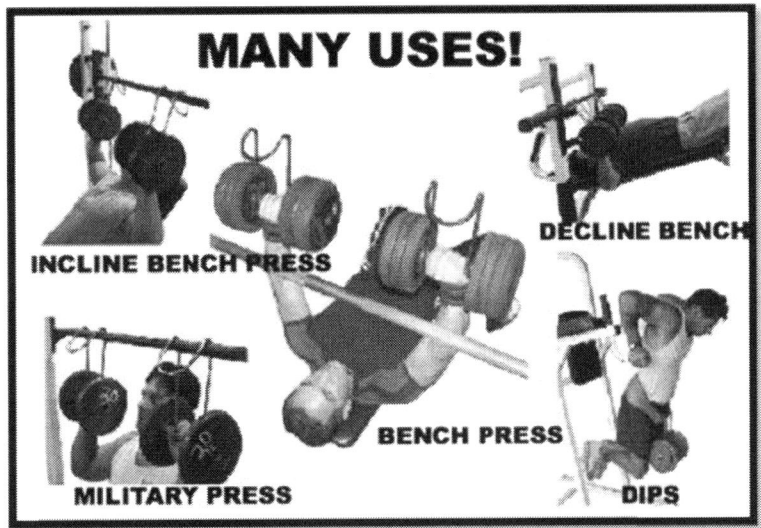

Made by New York Barbell of Elmira, New York, this simple hook device is easily retrofitted to fixed dumbbells or adjustable dumbbells for self-spotting or for weighted dips or pull-ups.

PowerBlock Dumbbells

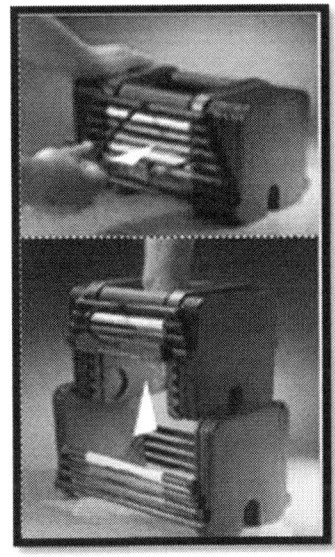

An early prototype of an adjustable dumbbell was first patented by David Shields, of Jacksonville, Florida, during the late 1980s. The PowerBlock consists of a fully adjustable (in 2.5-pound increments) set of cube-shaped dumbbells and stand. Putting the connected retainer pins in the desired holes easily adjusts the weight. There are some cool features that bear mention.

First, because there are four stabilizer bars spanning the two ends (with the padded handle in the middle of them), anyone can easily spot the user without having to hold the user's wrists or elbows. Simply hold onto one of the top stabilizer bars. That single feature, in and of itself, makes the PowerBlock safer than conventional dumbbells.

Next, with several sets of PowerBlocks in your commercial gym, all of the trainees can use the same amount of weight if they choose. No more waiting to do your set. They also take up far less space than a conventional rack of fixed dumbbells, can never be misplaced, and are considerably less expensive than a full set of fixed dumbbells. These are advantages in a well-equipped home gym as well. And, if they're inadvertently dropped (which has happens on occasion), they are very durable. For the trainee with limited time to put dumbbells together and limited space, but the desire to maximize results, PowerBlocks are the game changer!

Chapter IV: Forgotten Dumbbell Exercises

The inventor of the lead-shot-filled dumbbells and kettlebells was Professor Anthony Barker. In 1911, he marketed a wall poster course called "A Complete Course in Heavy Dumbell Exercises, To Obtain Strong, Healthy Muscles." Note that it's spelled with just one "b."

The chart included the startling necessity to wear a "well-made jock strap…to protect the back and the wall of the stomach, eliminating all dangers of strain or rupture." However, more startling was the array of dumbbell, kettlebell and barbell exercises the good professor chose to include in his course.

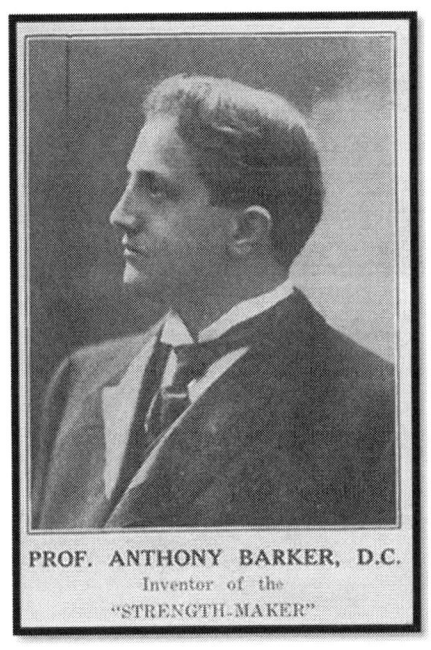

PROF. ANTHONY BARKER, D.C.
Inventor of the
"STRENGTH-MAKER"

Look at some of the unique dumbbell exercises that the professor's wall chart depicted. Some of these exercises have seen resurgence recently by "functional training" gurus. Like legendary strength coach Al Vermeil says, "You show me the exercise, I will show you what we used to call it."

Make no bones about it, each and every one of these movements requires tremendous stabilizer strength and control to execute, a feature sorely missing in the spandex and oil-clad, machine-infested gyms. Instead of showing off on the leg press, followthe great Vaudevillian Circus Strongman and give one of these exercises a shot. We have tried them with a weight that was as close to those depicted as we could get, and they were not duplicated by a couple of world-class strength athletes.

The Exercises

One-arm Dumbbell Bent Press (great for shoulders, triceps, and serratus anterior)

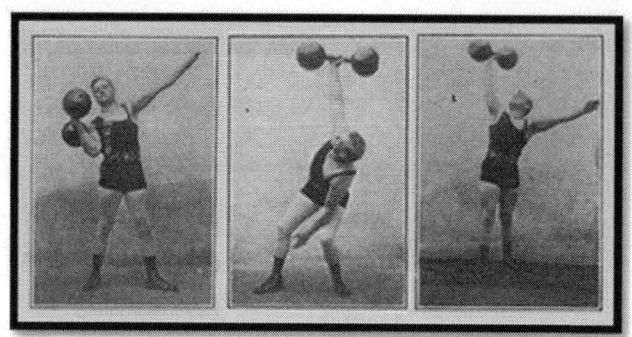

This was a staple of the old-time strongmen such as Eugene Sandow, Arthur Saxon, and Louis Cyr, but lost popularity because of potential risks posed by the contortion of the body and stresses placed on the shoulder, joint and spine. Like most difficult exercises, the bent press has long been branded "unsafe." Practitioners of the exercise are quick to point out that since it uses the leverage of the body to lift the weight, if done correctly, it can be quite safe.

Exercise Description

- Lift the dumbbell to either shoulder by a one- or two-handed clean, or by lifting one end and "rocking" it onto the shoulder. If using the right hand, which we are for this example, the right leg will be straight and directly underneath the weight, with the left leg bent at a slight angle. (Left hand is opposite.)

- Now, bend to the left, holding the weight in the same position. The bent position, hence the name "bent press," allows the arm to hold the weight in position without dropping down because of the body's leverage, creating an imaginary line between the bell and the floor that travels through the right arm and right leg.

- Next, continue to bend to the left until the arm is fully extended. The weight is not pressed, but held aloft while the body bends underneath it.

- To complete the lift, after the arm is fully extended, do a slight corkscrew to get underneath the weight in a half or full squat position, without pressing the weight. Once underneath the weight, with the arm locked out overhead holding the weight, stand up straight, still holding the weight overhead.

Legendary strongman pioneer Arthur Saxon holds the world record in the bent press with 371 pounds. Unofficially, reports surfaced of Saxon bent pressing 410 pounds.

Lying One-Arm Dumbbell Support, and Then Stand Up

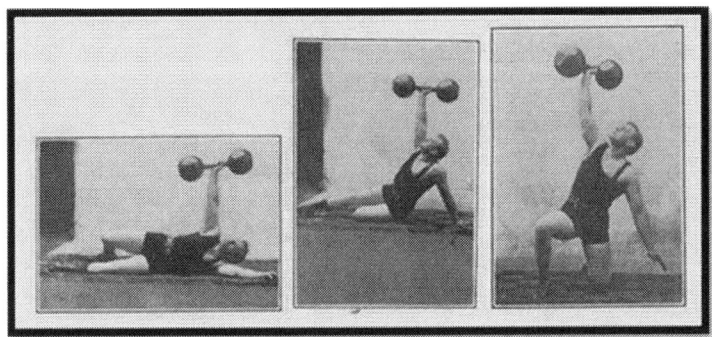

This is an unbelievable exercise in stability and control, let alone strength! Remember, show an old-timer an exercise and he will tell you what they used to call it. Yes, we are familiar with Turkish Get-Up but feel it's very important to pay homage to the pioneers.

Exercise Description

- Lie on the back with dumbbell in right hand held in extension

- Roll on to left side while the arm is held in extension

- Extend the left arm on the floor while resting on the hip, as seen in the photo

- Get on the left knee, like in photo 18, arm remains in extension

- Stand up to a fully erect position with arm held in extension

- Do opposite for left side

One-Arm Dumbbell Table Curls

For great arm development, we have to think past just modern-age, glossy muscle mags; these

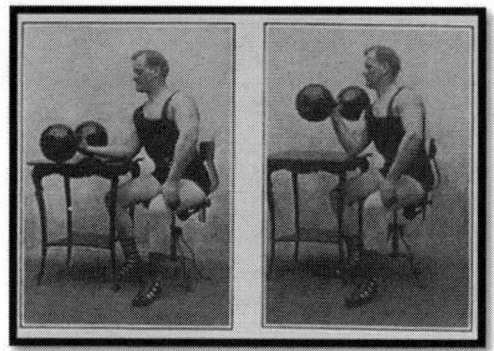

sources have some value, but so do the classics. Let's look to the heroes of old, in arm wrestling, to guys like the amazing Mac Batchelor. This exercise has cult-like allegiance amongst arm wrestlers! All you need is a dumbbell and a table. Make sure the table is sturdy.

The table curl is performed by placing your arm on a table or bench with a resting dumbbell in your hand. From this point, curl up toward your chest, and then repeat the motion by letting the dumbbell go back to the table as your arm stretches back to the starting position.

For arm wrestlers, the transfer to the table is huge because the movement simulates the pulling movement utilized in some arm wrestling techniques. Forearm and wrist strength is expedited by curling up and down on the table. You can take this a step further by grasping the dumbbell by the end of "bell" and every muscle in your forearms will cry "Uncle!"

Here is where an important distinction needs to be made—the starting point. For bodybuilding and general strength purposes, start this exercise at the end position with dumbbell at end range of flexion (touching shoulder or as close as mobility allows). From this point, lower the weight and perform the exercise repetitively. Why start from the top? You are a hell of a lot stronger eccentrically (negative) and on the downward movement, your muscles will store elastic-like energy that will assist in lifting the dumbbell back to the starting point. There is not a need to overcome dead weight by eliminating the stretch shortening cycle.

For the arm wrestler, overcoming dead weight is huge; starting from a bottom and top position is advised in training. His movement provides a hellacious overload for the top half of a curl; of course, we have to train the full range of motion for full development.

Next Bicep Work Try This Routine

- Table Curls for 4 sets of 6-10 reps as heavy as possible

- 1/2 rep—Incline Dumbbell Curls (bottom half only, emphasize stretch) 4 sets of 8-12 reps as heavy as possible

- Hammer Curls (Full Range of Motion) 3 sets of 12-15 reps as heavy as possible.

- Your biceps will be screaming!

Exercise Description

- Sit or stand at a table, and with elbow at chest level, grasp one dumbbell in hand

- Start with dumbbell in a full flexed elbow position

- From this position, lower dumbbell to table under control

- Forcefully curl dumbbell back to starting position

- Repeat

Ahrens Press

The largest mammoth of the early Muscle Beach era was the immortal Chuck Ahrens. Ahrens has been called everything from the reclusive power house to the mystery man. He was quiet, reserved and never would take off his shirt to pose for cameras. Ahrens preferred to do his 400-plus pound triceps extensions in a flannel shirt. In his prime, he weighed 330 pounds at 6 feet in height, with a non-expanded measurement of nearly 60 inches and 28-inch-wide shoulders. Ahrens was not just a mirage of meat either; he possessed superhuman strength! *Ironman Magazine* founder Perry Reader and other notable iron-game writers of the day all commented that he had the widest shoulder of any man alive.

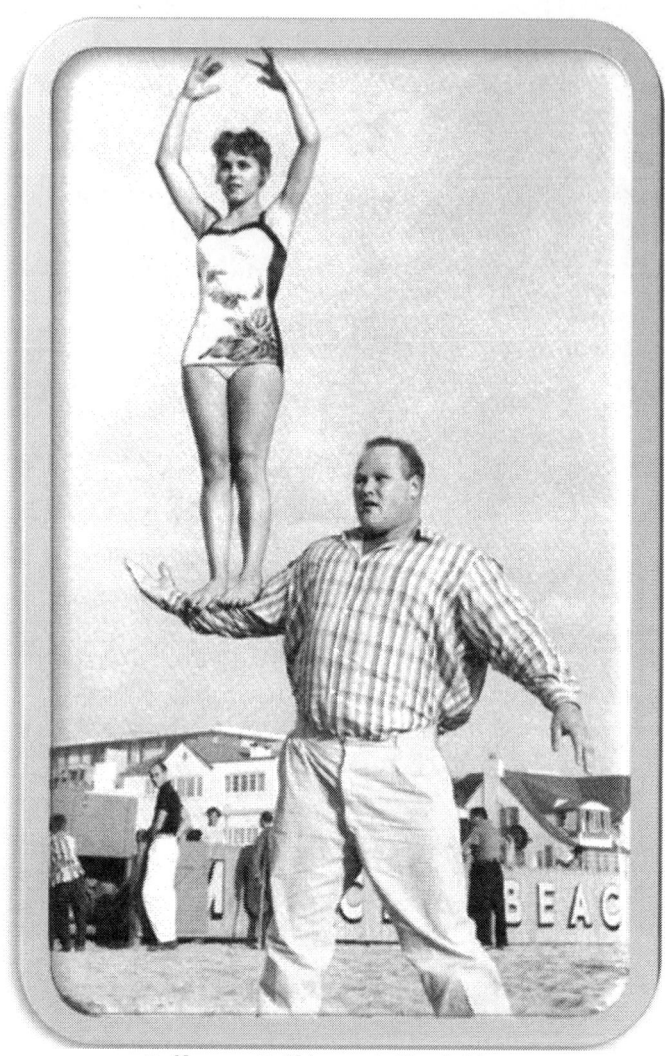

Half-man, Half-legend, Chuck Ahrens

Besides extremely heavy lateral raises and Herculean overhead barbell presses, many believe the superhuman deltoid development of Ahrens was catalyzed by a lift that is today affectionately known as the "Ahrens press."

The Ahrens press is a variation of the overhead dumbbell press, but instead of pressing the dumbbells straight up, you press them up and away laterally, sort of like making a V with both arms. Necessity was the mother of invention, in this case! Ahrens had no choice but to press the dumbbells in this style because he used special loadable dumbbells that were very long; in other words, it was impossible to press them straight because they would hit each other with the massive poundages he hoisted overhead.

For the bodybuilder, because of the lateral pressing motion, this exercise forces the medial delts or "caps" to work harder.

Exercise Description

- Grasp two dumbbells and lift them to shoulder level with a pronated grip

- From shoulder position, press the dumbbells out laterally (away from you)

- Finish with arms locked and at a 15- to 30-degree angle

- Return to starting position

Final Thoughts

It's not out with the old and in with new, and to answer Merle Haggard, the good times are not over for good. The key to success with dumbbell training is synergistically blending the most effective methods of the past with the newest innovations, using science as the guiding light.

Chapter V: Scientific Principles of Weight Training

The Perfectly-Developed Man

Professor Barker developed the chart below. When you compare the measurements of the "perfectly-developed man" of his day with those of today's bodybuilders, you will smile. But you will laugh out loud when you read the instructions for gaining and losing weight! We are borrowing many ideas from the old school but still ultimately refer to science as our guiding light.

Weights and Measurements of perfectly developed men

Height	Weight	Neck	Chest	Waist	Biceps	F'arms	Thighs	Calves
5 ft.	105 lbs.	11	32	28	11	9	15	11
5 " 1	110 "	11½	33	29	11½	9¼	16	11½
5 " 2	115 "	12	34	30	12	9½	17	12
5 " 3	120 "	12½	35	31	12½	10	18	12½
5 " 4	125 "	13	36	32	13	10¼	19	13
5 " 5	130 "	13½	37	33	13½	10¾	20	13½
5 " 6	135 "	14	38	34	14	11	21	14
5 " 7	145 "	14½	39	35	14½	11½	22	14½
5 " 8	150 "	15	40	36	15	12	23	15
5 " 9	160 "	15½	41	37	15½	12¼	24	15½
5 " 10	175 "	16	42	38	16	12½	25	16
5 " 11	185 "	16½	43	39	16½	13	26	16½
6 "	195 "	17	44	40	17	13½	27	17

IF YOU ARE OVERWEIGHT

Wear all wool heavy union suit and a heavy wool sweater on top of the union suit then exercise with the Strength-Maker dumbbells very quickly for ½ hour to 1 hour every day. When you bring your weight down to what it should be, then it is only necessary for you to exercise ½ hour every day.

IF YOU ARE UNDERWEIGHT

Put on as little clothes as possible with a strongly made jock strap and exercise with the Strength-Maker dumbbells ½ hour every day. Do each exercise very slowly. In a short time you will be able to develop enough healthy muscular tissue to bring your weight up to what it should be.

Let's take a look at the scientific principles guiding strength training.

Frequency, Intensity and Duration of Exercise

The darlings of late night infomercials may believe that dance moves, or whatever other snake oil they hawk, will solve the obesity epidemic, but remember, there is no magic potion or program—there are only principles.

Principles are universal laws. Adherence to principles results in the most favorable outcomes in training or life. There is no last-minute cramming like a college kid before an exam who wants to pass a class rather than truly receive an education. You reap what you sow; think of the law of the harvest. There are no shortcuts, but following principles allows the most direct path to exceeding your physical goals.

There are myriad definitions for the words "exercise" and "fitness." So, let's get straight to the point of each of these common words. Without "challenge" there is no exercise, and without exercise there can be no fitness. The key is that when you exercise—any form of exercise you choose to engage in—you *must* challenge your physical capabilities, and you must do it consistently. In so doing, your body will adapt to a higher and higher level of physical stress. This statement applies to weight training, running, stretching and all other forms of exercise!

Exercise vs. Training

If you're not challenging your physical ability, you are not exercising! You're just killing time or "maintaining." Furthermore, you need to be training, not just exercising. What's the difference? Exercise is performed for the effect it has today; training is performed with a long-term performance goal in mind. Feeling the burn, busting a sweat, doing an activity for its own sake or the feeling it immediately produces is exercise. Exercise is not bad! Remember, there is good, better and best when it comes to exercise. But we want the best, and that's why we are going to teach you how to train. By all means, however, always choose exercise over a sedentary lifestyle. Training is performed to reach a long-term performance goal, one that can be quantified. The series of acute adaptations over the course of the training cycle produces the long-term training adaptions or desired training effect. Improvement over time to meet a long-term goal is the objective of training. And you should remember this sage advice as you progress toward your training goal: No one has ever bench pressed 500 pounds raw and concurrently run a five-minute mile. Bottom line: You have one ass, so don't try and ride two horses!

Clearly Defining Training

"Getting fit" is not a goal; weighing a specific amount is. Achieving a specific amount of strength, body fat, or flexibility are all real goals that can be achieved with training.

Training is long term; exercise is immediate. Many folks are not competitive athletes but can benefit from a training regimen. And, yes, this also applies to dumbbell training!

Bear in mind that the challenge that you impose upon your muscles must be in small increments, easy at first and gradually—over weeks and months of time—increasing in intensity. Now you know that challenge relates to intensity. If the weight you're using doesn't challenge you, it's not heavy enough. Putting it another way, if you're training at an intensity level that's too low for you, amp up the intensity!

Story of Milo

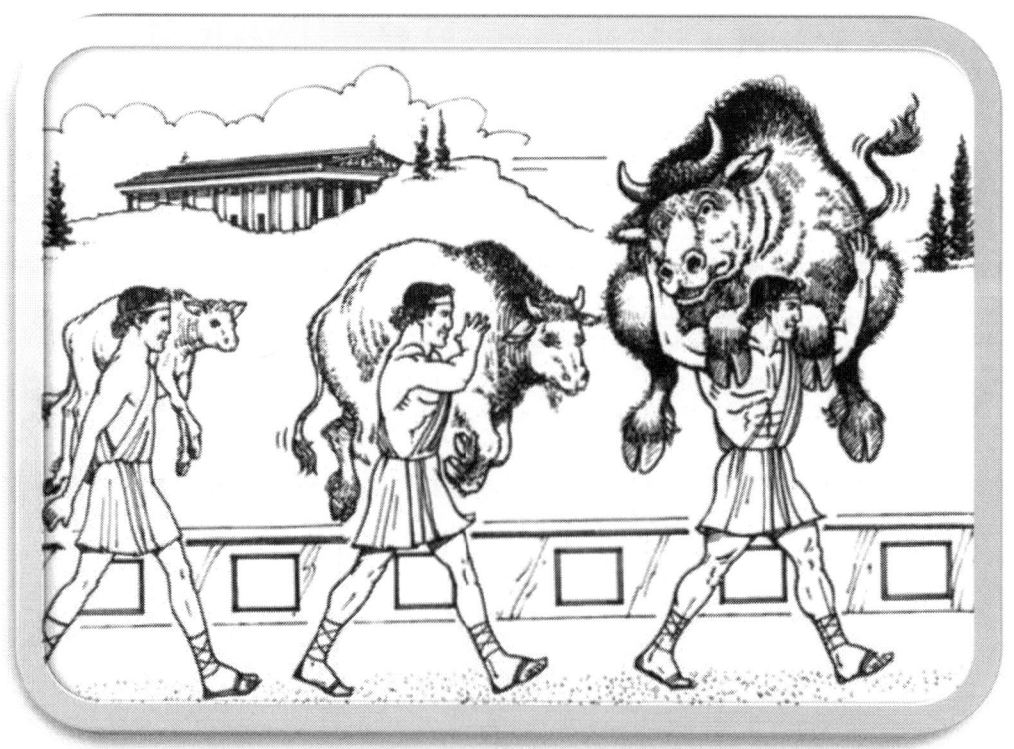

Milo of Croton was a wrestler with several ancient Olympic titles under his belt, considered by most historians to have been the greatest wrestler of antiquity. His heyday was the sixth century B.C., but to this day, his name is associated with strength. Milo built his strength by using progressive overload before it was a categorized as a Granddaddy Law or principle at all.

Milo had a baby bull or a calf; Milo lifted that calf every single day, and as the calf grew bigger, Milo became stronger. Milo did this all the way until the calf was a full-grown bull and then he was the strongest man in the world. Milo eventually carried the adult bull on his shoulders around the Coliseum.

Milo started small, used micro progressions daily and became the strongest man in the world. Progressive overload worked then and it works now.

The law of overload is one of the first principles learned in exercise physiology. It means: Mother Nature overcompensates for training stress by giving you bigger and stronger muscles. No resistance training program will be successful without progressive overload at its foundation.

Overload Misapplied

It's common to hear, "If something is working well, don't change a thing." If training is going well now, this mindset will halt progress in a New York minute.

Changing something means intensifying training and this has been bastardized to the umpteenth degree. Think of all the crazy exercises like doing squats on bosu balls; if you're an alpine skier, we can see the rationale. But if the objective is to get stronger or gain size, that's downright stupid and dangerous. Science and common sense concur.

Unfortunately, at the expense of results, celebrity trainers perpetuated entertainment over what works in order to keep clients interested; maybe they are hoping since Coney Island was put on the map by bizarre tricks, they can follow suit. They should realize their clients will stay interested if they help them get great results with what's proven to work.

Think about it. If you constantly change things and totally randomize your training, how in the hell will you continually overload? It's as logical as the temperance society inviting Popcorn Sutton to give a speech.

Overloading needs some sort of quantitative assessment.

Progressive Overload Misapplied

Overloading your training is not just our opinion, it's a Granddaddy Law. We don't make the rules. Many times the bizarre "functional training" realm will dismiss progressive overload with randomization. After all, why squat when you can do one-legged occluded goblet squats on a trampoline holding a kettlebell overhead?

The bodybuilding crowd will attempt to dismiss progressive overload with constantly changing exercises for "confusion." Because of the repeated bout effect, this logic has more validity than the functional training crowd's charades, but misapplication was seen recently when a pro bodybuilder was having clients do leg presses with sliders on the leg press to activate different parts of the quad. For the bodybuilder, more frequent exercise rotation is needed but when cycling exercises, you need to overload them from when you performed them last. Keeping a training journal makes this simple.

Progressive Overload Outdated?

A few prominent strength coaches have talked about progressive overload being outdated, which is downright silly. If you do not constantly overload your training, you will not get stronger. Their idea is that if someone bench pressed the bar today and improved five pounds a week for three years, they would bench press 825 pounds, 103 pounds over the most weight ever bench pressed.

But linear progression without deloads, using the exact same rep scheme and set scheme, will run someone into a wall. Mel Siff, elaborating on the great Soviet sports scientist Yuri Verkoshansky, offered a solution with what he called periods of increased loading, in essence, cycling training. You do a 12-week linear cycle by gradually decreasing reps; every time you use eight reps, use more weight than last time with eight reps.

Westside barbell uses progressive overload. Think about it. By rotating a ton of specialty exercises, let's say for a max effort squat or deadlift, one does safety box squats off a 14-inch box for a max double, and the objective is to beat the record set last time. Say this exercise was last performed six months ago with 405 for a max double, then it better be 406 or more now. Any system that is effective at building strength progressively overloads. Training, meaning working toward a long-term goal with purpose and long-term adaptations in mind, requires progressive overload. Remove progressive overload and you are working out. This means exercising for an immediate feeling. Working out is fine to slightly improve health, but if you have the slightest desire to take this to the next level, training is required.

Progressive Overload Applied to Dumbbell Training

Since we cannot just continue to pile weight on the bar without stalling out, let's explore seven alternative options to overload training.

1. **Load (resistance) increases**—This is the most obvious way. Don't think in terms of 10-pound dumbbell jumps. You can buy one-pound magnetic dumbbells plates online, so don't be like bodybuilders with small IQs and big egos.

2. **Increase volume**—Simply do more. This could be an increase in the amount of sets performed, weight lifted, or repetitions performed. Volume is (sets × × rep × × weight lifted). Do not do this with light weights under 65 percent of a one-rep max. Obviously, dumbbell bench pressing 100 pounds for 10 sets of 10 provides a different training effect than dumbbell bench pressing 500 for 10 sets of 2 reps, although both are 10,000 pounds of volume.

3. **Increase range of motion**—Doing a snatch grip deadlift with 75 percent of a one-rep max deadlift is much more difficult than a regular deadlift. Try dumbbell deadlifts off the floor over barbell deadlifts or deep dumbbell bench presses over barbell presses. Dumbbells allow more free movement and make it much easier to increase range of motion.

4. **Alter repetition speed**—Slow down the eccentric and prolong time under tension; speed up the concentric and take force production to a whole new level.

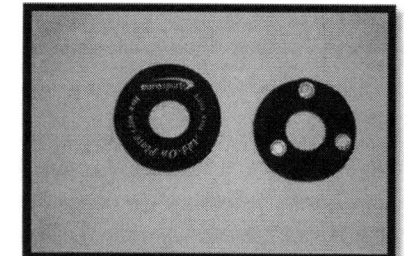

5. **Shorten rest intervals**—Do the same amount of work in less time or do more work in the same amount of time. Both increase training density, a legitimate way to overload training.

6. **Change exercises**—More frequent changes in exercises are needed when hypertrophy is the objective, but pure strength accessory exercises can be changed every couple blocks.

7. **Increase frequency**—Train more often.

The idea is to load linearly as long as possible, then start pulling more tricks out of the hat as you journey from beginner to intermediate, then to advanced training status.

Consistency

Consistency is key. "How often should I train?" The simple answer is always going to be "consistently." Don't miss workouts!

Let's say you train 20 days a month, five days a week. Every other week, you miss one workout. Most people think that's good, but IT SUCKS! You are missing 10 percent of your workouts! If you work 250 days a year, yet miss 25 days of work yearly, you will receive a pink slip in record time.

When you train, every workout has purpose; every workout builds on the previous one. Missing workouts throws everything out of whack. Don't do it. Training thrice weekly consistently trumps four or five times sporadically.

Frequency Guidelines

Another simple rule of thumb followed for years is to hit each muscle or muscle group three times a week. We reject this simplistic approach because:

- Some muscles require more time than others for complete recovery.
- The more explosive you are in moving the weight, the more time you require for recovery.
- Lowering heavy weights slowly increases your need for recovery because of the slight damage done to the muscle cells in controlling the descent of the weight and increased time under tension.
- Applying maximum intensity in your training efforts may require a longer recovery period.

- External factors, such as sleep patterns and nutritional status, weigh on your recovery time.

- Women take a bit longer to recover than men.

- Aging slows the recovery process.

Bottom line: All these things show clearly how this Dark Age notion is in grave violation of the Principle of Individual Differences.

The Most Effective System for You

The following chart will be helpful in establishing the most effective training program for you personally.

We have provided sample dumbbell workouts later in this book, as well as a discourse on training systems.

Training to Individual Needs

"I can pass by the weight room, smell the iron inside, and instantly begin to grow," might say someone who thrives on very little exercise, while others seem to be incapable of making gains no matter how hard, long and frequently they train. This is referred to as one's "tolerance to exercise," a term coined by Arthur Jones years ago.

One's "tolerance" is high if more exercise is needed, and low if less is needed. There are many variables that can affect your exercise tolerance. Of course, genetics ranks highest on the list below, and you'll notice several such factors. Others, on the other hand, are able to be manipulated in various ways.

- Red vs. white muscle fiber ratio
- Tolerance of pain
- Level of "psych"
- Amount of rest since last workout

- Perceived exertion
- Amount of eccentric stress (which causes connective tissue microtrauma)
- Incentive level
- Strength-to-weight ratio
- Time of last meal (energy)
- Type of foods eaten at last meal (glycemic index)
- Use of ergogenic techniques or substances
- Musculoskeletal leverage factors
- Motor unit recruitment capabilities
- Skill level at exercise being performed (if such is required, e.g., cleans)
- Equipment quality and design
- Environmental factors (e.g., heat, cold, etc.)
- Size of muscle being exercised
- Various intra- and extracellular biochemical factors
- How close you are to your maximum potential in size or strength
- The use of banned drugs such as anabolic steroids (we *do not* condone their use!)

All these factors, and perhaps several more as yet undreamed of, will affect how frequently you should train each body part and how best to split your routine.

Fast Gainers, Slow Gainers and In Between

Several years ago, after chatting with Arthur and reading some of his thinking on the topic, Fred began charting other lifters' reps at 80 percent max. He found that guys who were so-called "fast" gainers were only able to do four to six reps at 80 percent, while lifters who seemingly never made great gains were able to rep out at around 15-20 reps with 80 percent of their max. Apparently, so-called "fast gainers" have rather poor anaerobic strength endurance. This is explainable, in part, by the fact that they probably have mostly white muscle fiber, which has fast twitch/low oxidative capabilities. Conversely, slow gainers are probably mostly red muscle fiber (slow twitch/high oxidative) and therefore may possess greater ability for rapid during-set recovery.

The problem is, however, that each muscle group's tolerance of exercise probably differs. Each exercise you do for each body part can—and often does—possess an entirely individual rep ability at 80 percent max. To discern your specific tolerance level for each body part, follow these simple instructions:

1. Determine your approximate one-repetition maximum (1RM) for each exercise.

2. Load 80 percent on the bar (machine) and rep out with it for one all-out effort to see how many reps you can do. Testing is recommended on a barbell or machine, and results will carry over to dumbbells.

3. Apply this information to the table below to determine each body part's exercise tolerance.

4. Take into account *all* of the factors listed above that can affect your exercise tolerance.

5. Critically evaluate whether your predicted exercise tolerance levels stand up to what you know from experience to be true. Remember, "low tolerance" means that you probably make easy gains for that body part, and "high tolerance" means that you're probably a hard gainer for that body part.

Here is an example of what we've found in regards to exercise tolerances for fast gainers, average gainers and slow gainers. Perhaps you'll find these figures to be pretty close estimates. But perhaps you won't. One thing is clear: You must look! Your continued progress toward your maximum potential may well depend on it!

Exercise Tolerance Chart

Reps Performed with 80 percent Max	Standard Deviation from Mean	Tolerance Level	Ability to Make Gains
4 or less	−3	Very, very low	Fast Gainer (20 percent–25 percent of total population)
4–6	−2	Very low	
6–10	−1	Low	
10–13	Mean	Average	Average Gainer (50–60 percent of total population)
13–17	+1	High	Slow Gainer (20–25 percent of total population)
17–21	+2	Very high	
21 or more	+3	Very, very high	

Slow Gainers (Usually predominately red muscle fiber)

Days of Recovery Required for Each Body Part Before Training It Again

	Days of Rest "Light Day"	Days of Rest "Medium Day"	Days of Rest "Heavy Day"
Large Muscle Groups: • Upper Legs • Lower Back	3	4	5
Medium Size Muscle Groups: • Chest • Upper Back • Biceps • Triceps • Shoulders	2	3	4
Smaller Muscle Groups: • Midsection • Calves • Forearms	1	2	3

Slow Gainers often benefit from 10 or more sets of 15-20 reps

Average Gainers (usually a mix of red and white muscle fiber)
Days of Recovery Required for Each Body Part before Training it Again

	Days of Rest "Light Day"	Days of Rest "Medium Day"	Days of Rest "Heavy Day"
Large Muscle Groups: • Upper Legs • Lower Back	4	5	6
Medium Size Muscle Groups: • Chest • Upper Back • Biceps • Triceps • Shoulders	3	4	5
Smaller Muscle Groups: • Midsection • Calves • Forearms	2	3	4

Average gainers often benefit most from 5-8 sets of 10-12 reps

Fast Gainers (usually predominantly white muscle fiber)
Days of Recovery Required for Each Body Part before Training it Again

	Days of Rest "Light Day"	Days of Rest "Medium Day"	Days of Rest "Heavy Day"
Large Muscle Groups: • Upper Legs • Lower Back	5	6	7
Medium Size Muscle Groups: • Chest • Upper Back • Biceps • Triceps • Shoulders	4	5	6
Smaller Muscle Groups: • Midsection • Calves • Forearms	3	4	5

Fast gainers often benefit most from three to five sets of four to eight reps done explosively.

By critically evaluating your individual muscles' tolerance to exercise, you can more easily "fine tune" your training regimen to provide maximum gains in the shortest possible time. But don't forget the other factors that may affect your recovery rate. Look at the list again (above). How have you accounted for the effect of each of these variables on your progress? Have you raised or lowered your reps and sets accordingly? Have you increased or decreased the frequency of your workouts commensurably? Have you increased training intensity? Have you taken into account your ratio of white versus red fiber and adjusted your exercise load and movement speed accordingly?

Why Can't You Just Copy The Pros?

Why is it that most newcomers to bodybuilding, and even most intermediate-level bodybuilders, can't make continued gains using a split they copied from one of the pros? It's quite simple, really.

First of all, you must be truthful with yourself in answering some basic questions.

Are you as fastidious as the pro you seek to emulate in all that you do? Your supplement schedule? Your use of anabolic or ergogenic aids? Your diet? Have you as much time "in the trenches" as the pro? How long have you been forcing your body to adapt to stress?

Most pros have forced adaptations to their muscles and other bodily systems that have taken years to accomplish. As your body changes over time, your susceptibility to further change does as well. New forms of stress force different adaptive processes to occur, and each adaptation requires different stressors and training schedules in order to take your body one more step closer to its maximum potential.

So as you change your body, your body demands different scheduling for further adaptation to take place. It isn't simply a matter of piling on more pig iron to satisfy the progressive overload principle. It's more complicated than that. One of the biggest mistakes serious weight trainees tend to make is that they do not build their programs with this important fact in mind.

As you change, so must your training because your body's "tolerance" to that level or type of stress has changed. And how you split your training can be an important source of new adaptive stress to which you have not yet adapted.

Gainer Variability

Most of you are not "hard gainers" or "fast gainers" in all body parts. Further, as you get closer to your maximum potential—where all professional bodybuilders and powerlifters are—you may become a hard gainer, whereas earlier in your career your gains seemed to come easy. Or maybe you've remained an easy gainer but have yet to discover the type of stress your body now requires to force continued growth.

Through experimentation, we assure you that finding your own level of "tolerance" (body part per body part) will make a big difference. Where to begin? Here are a few examples of how you can split your training program. Adjust them at will.

Examples Of Three Days Per Week Single Split Training Programs For Easy Gainers:
(Monday, Wednesday, Saturday)

	M	T	W	T	F	S	S	M	T	W	T	F	S	S	M	T	W	T
Upper Legs	H							M					L				M	
Lower Back	H							M					L				M	
Chest			L			M		H					M		L			
Upper Back			L			M		H					M		L			
Biceps	L		M			H				M			L			H		
Triceps	L		M			H				M			L			H		
Shoulders			H			M		L		M			H				M	
Midsection	M		H			M		M		H			M		M		H	
Calfs	M		H			M		M		H			M		M		H	
Forearms	M		H			M		M		H			M		M		H	

Example Of Four Days Per Week Single Split Training Programs For Easy Gainers:
(Monday, Tuesday, Thursday, Saturday)

	M	T	W	T	F	S	S	M	T	W	T	F	S	S	M	T	W	T
Upper Legs	H							M					L			M		
Lower Back	H							M					L			M		
Chest		L		M				H					M			L		M
Upper Back		L		M				H					M			L		M
Biceps	M			H				M			L		M			H		
Triceps	M			H				M			L		M			H		
Shoulders																		
Midsection	M			H				M			H					M		H
Calfs		H				M			H				M			H		
Forearms		H				M			H				M			H		

Example Of Five Days Per Week Single Split Training Programs For Easy Gainers:
(Weekends Off):

	M	T	W	T	F	S	S	M	T	W	T	F	S	S	M	T	W	T
Upper Legs	H							M				L				M		
Lower Back	H							M				L				M		
Chest		L		M				H				M				L		M
Upper Back		L		M				H				M				L		M
Biceps	M		H					M		L		M				H		
Triceps	M		H					M		L		M				H		
Shoulders		M			H					M		L			M		H	
Midsection																		
Calfs	L		M		H					M		L			M		H	
Forearms	L		M		H					M		L			M		H	

Example Of Six Days Per Week Single Split Training Programs For Average Gainers:
(Sunday Off):

	M	T	W	T	F	S	S	M	T	W	T	F	S	S	M	T	W	T
Upper Legs	H					M				L			M				H	
Lower Back	L					M				H			M				L	
Chest			L			M		H					M		L			
Upper Back			L			M		H					M		L			
Biceps	M			H				M			L				M			H
Triceps	M			H				M			L				M			H
Shoulders		M			H					M			L			M		H
Midsection				M		H							M				H	
Calfs		H			M			H				M				H		
Forearms		H			M			H				M				H		

Examples Of Three Day Double Split Training Programs For Average Gainers:

Monday Wednesday and Saturday:

		M	T	W	T	F	S	S	M	T	W	T	F	S	S	M	T	W	T
Upper Legs	1	H							M					L				M	
	2																		
Lower Back	1																		
	2	H							M					L				M	
Chest	1			L			M		H					M		L			
	2																		
Upper Back	1																		
	2			L			M		H					M		L			
Biceps	1	L		M			H				M			L		H			
	2																		
Triceps	1																		
	2	L		M			H				M			L		H			
Shoulders	1			H			M		L		M			H				M	
	2																		
Midsection	1	M		H			M		M		H			M		M		H	
	2																		
Calfs	1																		
	2	M		H			M		M		H			M		M		H	
Forearms	1	M		H			M		M		H			M		M		H	
	2																		

	M	T	W	T	F	S	S	M	T	W	T	F	S	S	M	T	W	T
Upper Legs	H					M				L			M				H	
Lower Back	L					M				H			M				L	
Chest			L			M		H					M		L			
Upper Back			L			M		H					M		L			
Biceps	M			H					M			L			M			H
Triceps	M			H					M			L			M			H
Shoulders		M			H					M			L			M		
Midsection				M				H					M				H	
Calfs		H			M				H			M				H		
Forearms		H			M				H			M				H		

Examples Of Four Day Double Split Training Programs For Average Gainers:
Monday, Tuesday, Thursday, Saturday:

		M	T	W	T	F	S	S	M	T	W	T	F	S	S	M	T	W	T
Upper Legs	1																		
	2	H					M		L					M					H
Lower Back	1	H					M		L					M					H
	2																		
Chest	1		L				M	H						M			L		
	2		L				M	H						M			L		
Upper Back	1																		
	2		L				M	H						M	L				
Biceps	1	M			H					M		L				M			H
	2																		
Triceps	1																		
	2	M			H					M		L				M			H
Shoulders	1																		
	2																		
Midsection	1																		
	2			M				H						M			H		
Calfs	1		H				M		H					M			H		
	2		H				M		H					M			H		
Forearms	1		H				M		H					M			H		
	2																		

That was in depth look, if you really want to "train" and fine tune this sucker. For the

intermediate trainee, the below chart is a good starting guideline.

Body Part	Days of Rest After Easy Workouts	Days of Rest After Moderately Intense Workouts	Days of Rest After Highly Intense Workouts
Chest	2	3	4
Shoulders	2	3	4
Trapezius	3	4	5
Lower Back	3	4	5
Upper Back	2	3	4
Biceps	2	3	4
Triceps	2	3	4
Abdominals	1	2	3
Quadriceps	3	4	5
Hamstrings	3	4	5
Calves	1	2	3
Forearms	1	2	3

Final Thoughts

You are not the master of your own destiny, principles are! By adhering to these universal laws, you can ultimately determine your training fate. You now have the tools to custom tailor a training program to your needs.

Above all else remember: **consistency + overload= synergy**.

Chapter VI: Advantages of Dumbbell Training

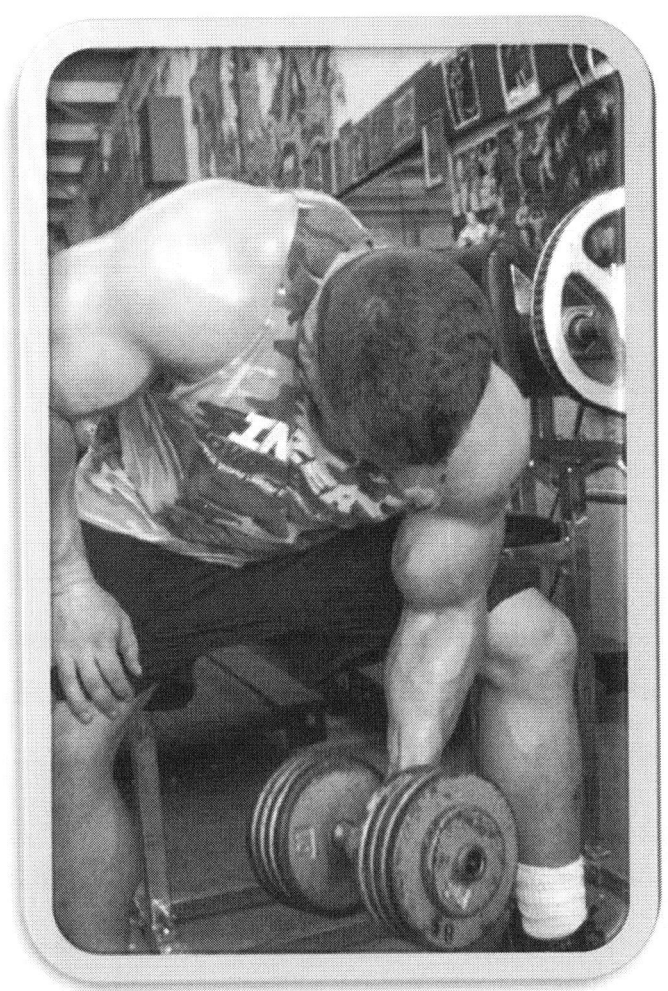

Co-author Josh Bryant

Don't worry about the latest trending topic on Twitter or updating your Facebook status at the gym; the tools you are given in this book will make it obvious you are hammering the pig iron.

Be Careful

The injury rate in commercial gyms is higher around the dumbbell rack than anywhere else in the gym, not so much from improper exercise technique (although this factor certainly can be a problem) as from dropped weights, tripping, distractions, bumping caused by passers-by, and improper cradling of dumbbells on the rack. Applying a bit of common sense and focusing on what's going on around you render these hazards insignificant.

Dumbbell Training vs. Machine Training

1. Because you're constantly forced to adjust and readjust the position of the dumbbells, synergistic (helping) muscles and stabilizer muscles act more prominently, overall strength is improved, and you are a bit more "injury-proofed." This is because the "weak link" muscles in various movements are strengthened more easily and thoroughly with dumbbells.

2. Dumbbell exercises can be tailored easily to more closely match the neurological patterns of sports skills owing to improved joint kinesthesis (position awareness), leverage similarities and total body involvement. Machines force one to succumb to preset motor patterns, set to the "average" user. What the hell is average anyway?

3. Dumbbells are more versatile than machines or barbells. Any movement can be done with dumbbells, whereas machines restrict you to their movement, and barbells typically require symmetrical movement between left and right sides. Dumbbells help one identify and correct imbalances between limbs.

4. A set of adjustable dumbbells (e.g., the PowerBlock dumbbells or adjustable dumbbells) is less expensive and takes up less space than other home gym machines, making it ideal for home gyms as well as for commercial gyms.

5. No time, no space, no problem! Minimalist training programs have soared in popularity over the past decade, and dumbbells are the ultimate minimalist training tool. A holistic bodybuilding workout can be accomplished in a walk-in closet.

6. You can train alone! Spotting is literally life or death on many barbell exercises. With dumbbells, it's a luxury, not a necessity.

Safety and Efficiency in Dumbbell Training is a Must

1. Because smaller synergists and stabilizer muscles are more prominently targeted with dumbbells than with machines or barbells, they tend to fatigue before the prime mover(s), and control of the dumbbells is easily lost.

2. Dumbbells with free plates and removable collars can come apart if care is not taken to tightly secure the collars, so check them before each set.

3. Adjustments in weight require affixing or removing plates and collars—often a time-consuming and tedious ordeal. Clearly, this speaks well for having either an entire rack of fixed dumbbells or a PowerBlock set. (But if you are training at home you are saving time by cutting out a commute both ways and not having yuppies on cell phones hoggin' all the "bells.")

4. Going up and down the rack trying to find the right weights is a common and exasperating experience in most gyms, so put the dumbbells back in their proper order when you've completed your set. Waiting for someone to finish with the set of dumbbells you need in order to continue your workout is also a problem at many gyms. Gather dumbbells ahead of time. This is not an exercise in Dale Carnegie's *How to Win Friends and Influence People*; act more like Attila the Hun. You need an open, clutter-free space to use dumbbells. It can be hazardous for large groups of unorganized or inexperienced people to use dumbbells in a small area. So keep a sharp, peripheral perspective for wayward passers-by or training paraphernalia lying around on the floor.

Spotting Dumbbell Exercises

The most common spotting technique for dumbbells (dumbbell bench press, incline press, and military press) is to cradle the elbow and provide assistance from there. Excellent, experienced spotters can use the technique effectively as they follow the natural curve of the lifter's plane of movement (positively adding to and not adversely affecting the lifter's movement), and many lifters prefer to be spotted with this method.

However, we said, "experienced spotter"; most spotters do not fall into this category, thereby making cradling the elbow one of the most dangerous forms of spotting dumbbell exercises. It may even be more dangerous than having no spotter at all! At least without spotters, it's easy to dump the dumbbells.

Push the elbow and the elbow moves toward the body. If the elbow isn't extending while you push the elbow, the weight goes toward the body as well and eventually falls on the lifter! Not a safe technique, is it?

For most spotters, grabbing the wrists of the lifter near the dumbbell is a safer spotting alternative. On exercises like dumbbell pullovers, which require both hands grasping the dumbbell, spot the lower half of the dumbbell (closest to the floor).

Problems with Machine Training

Dr. Pat O'Shea, author of the first college text ever written on weight training (*Scientific Principles and Methods of Strength Fitness,* Addison-Wesley Publishing Company, 1976), elaborated on the benefits of free weight training versus machine training. He listed "10 perils of machine training":

1. No machine can provide full-range, multiple-joint movements as closely as free weights. Dumbbells are superior to barbells; barbells are superior to machines.

2. Motor skill engrams aren't established with machines as well as free weights. Theoretically, regression can happen switching from free weights to machines.

3. The carry-over value of free weight training is superior to that provided by machine training.

4. Machine training won't help you develop a high level of fluid, dynamic full range of motion and athletic strength.

5. The body is a homogeneous unit that engages in ballistic movements, particularly those generated by strong hip thrust.

6. Machine training doesn't provide for training variety and variability.

7. Machines don't permit the mind and body to develop in synchronization.

8. Machine training does not stress the psycho-endocrine systems.

9. Machine training does not provide for positive training experience.

10. Machine training does not provide for continuous long-term motivation.

These 10 points are elaborated on in the legendary *Power: A Scientific Approach* (Contemporary Books, 1989). They explain, in large part, why so many people fail to get themselves in peak condition if all they do is train with machines. They also explain why people get injured so much: Moving through prescribed patterns and ranges of motion just isn't the way the good Lord intended for you to move!

Dumbbells are Functional Training

We have only hinted at the one important point that needs to be addressed. It brings us even closer in understanding the injuries and drop-out rates. The simple fact is that, with the use of machines, you're almost always sitting, lying or leaning. Why? The pussification of modern humanity!

Overweight soccer moms and corporate softies just want to "exercise" and want the path of least resistance; unfortunately, the road to hell is paved with good intentions and that's the path of least results. Sitting is easy, lying down is easy, just like leaning on a machine.

PT Barnum/L. Ron Hubbard Model

You have to wonder why some proponents of circuit training set up machines in this manner: Simple adherence to the PT Barnum philosophy of "there is a sucker born every minute," or the L. Ron Hubbard philosophy of "the best way to make a million dollars is start a religion," i.e., Arthur Jones and his "disciples." Plain and simple, it's dollar-driven; results take a back seat.

Injury Rates

The chances of injury, both during and as a result of training on machines, is far greater than when lifting free weights and standing on your own two feet. Admittedly, this seems odd. Most of us assume that machines offer the user a bit more safety than free weights. You know, limited range of movement, carefully hidden moving parts, total lack of ballistic stress, no stability requirements and so forth.

Not so according to the literature:

- Weightlifters have less than half the injury rate per 100 hours of training than do those engaged in other forms of weight training: 17 vs. 35. (Hamill, B. Relative Safety of Weightlifting and Weight Training. Journal of Strength and Conditioning Research, 8(1):53-57. 1994)

- Retired Olympic weightlifters had lower lifetime incidence and prevalence of low back pain than a control group of normal active men of similar age; 23 percent vs. 31 percent. (Granhed, H. et al. Low back pain among retired wrestlers and heavyweight lifters. The American Journal of Sports Medicine, 16(5):530-533. 1988)

- Mike Stone, et al, provided an excellent review of the research literature on this topic. The inescapable conclusion was that weightlifting (free weights) is indeed the safest method of weight training. (Stone, M. H., A. C. Fry, M. Ritchie, L. Stoessel-Ross, and J. L. Marsit. Injury potential and safety aspects of weightlifting movements. Strength and Conditioning. June: 15-21. 1994).

Wisdom of O'Shea

It is clear now that Dr. O'Shea knew what he was taking about. The very forms of stress that machines force you to avoid are the ones that produce the desired training adaptations, because they simulate how we move about Planet Earth.

How Can I Make Dumbbells Safer and More Effective Than Machine Training?

The answer to this innocent question is that they already are! Scientific research says it quite clearly. On the other hand, it would be irresponsible to not leave these few points of caution. You will not experience the benefits of dumbbell training unless you know a few things to avoid:

- Poor technique in executing the movement (placing too much stress on connective tissues and the smaller synergists or stabilizers by getting out of the "groove")

- Premature use of an intense training method (going ballistic before a solid foundation is developed, i.e. rest-pausing, mechanical advantage drop sets or any other advanced bodybuilding technique)

- Improper frame of mind while lifting (lack of focus, intensity, dedication, not tweeting, texting or bird-doggin' the opposite sex while training—have a definitive purpose)

- Repeating a movement until fatigue forces you to fail (predisposition to focus problems as well as injury)

This last technique can benefit an advanced bodybuilder in the acquisition of hypertrophy, but with its higher reward, there is a higher risk.

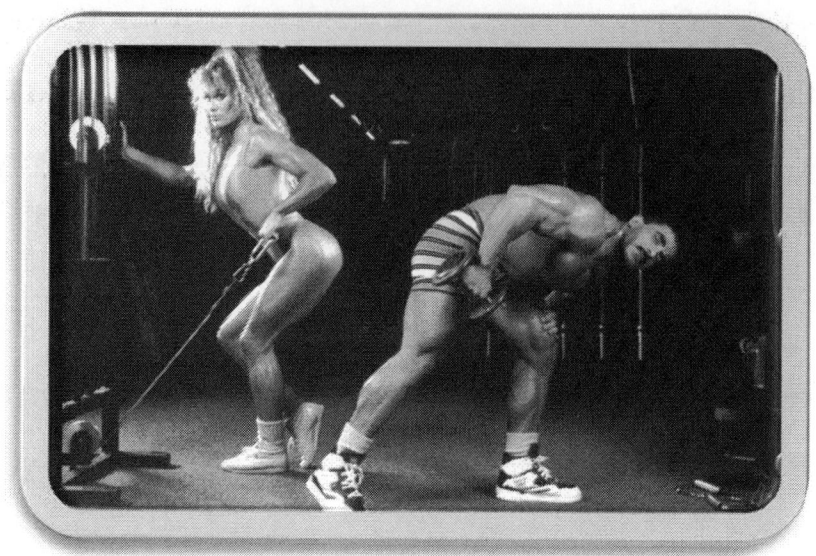

Should I Abandon Machines?

Absolutely not! After all, if you use them correctly, some machines can be quite effective.

Further, some machines allow movements that you cannot perform with dumbbells. Just expand your horizons a bit!

Chapter VII: Systems of Training

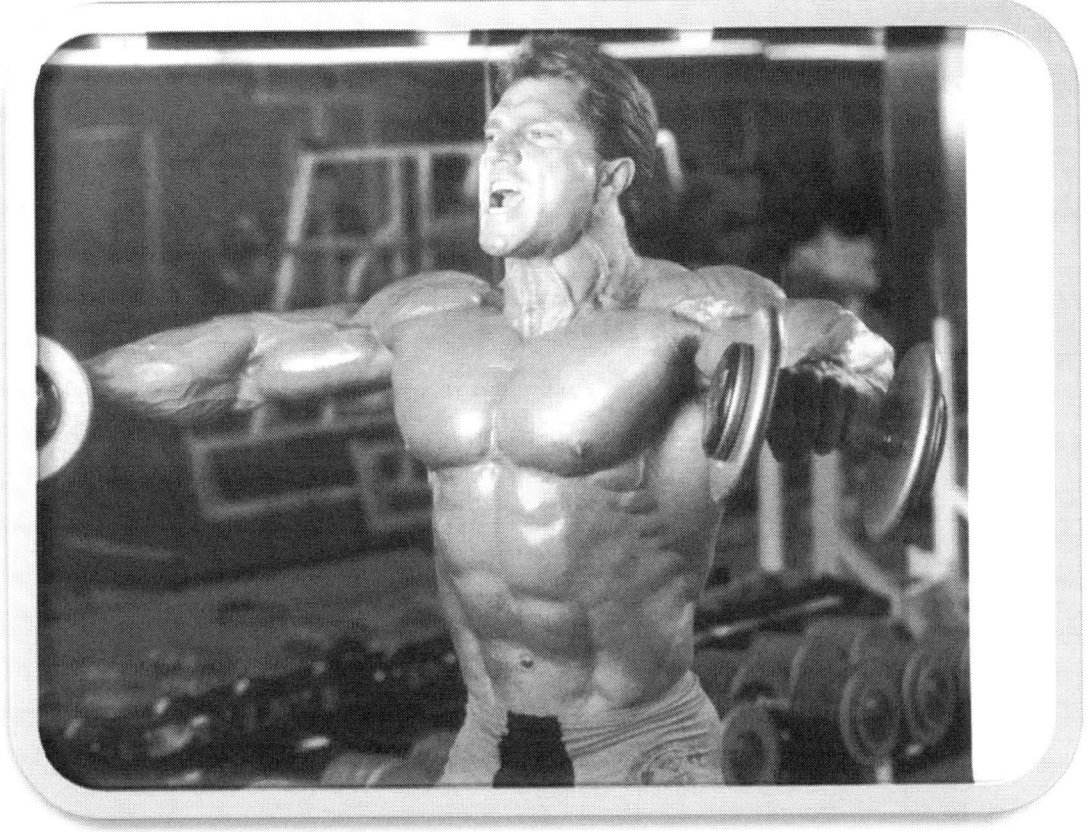

Gary Strydom, destroying the delts with dumbbells

A VERY practical definition of fitness is your ability to meet the exigencies of your lifestyle with ease—and room to spare for life's little emergencies. What constitutes fitness for one person isn't necessarily fitness for another. Laborers need a different level of fitness than do office workers because the demands of their lifestyles are different. Coaches need not be as fit as the athletes they train, generals needn't be as fit as the soldiers they command, and older adults require a different set of standards for lifestyle fitness than do younger adults.

With that, here is one small, but important, piece of wisdom. Regardless of your fitness goals, the fastest, most efficient, and safest way to accomplish them is going to include free weight training. And it behooves you to know a bit about some of the more effective weight training systems before you begin.

The Set System

The set system is perhaps the single most popular system in use. This is so for athletes, fitness enthusiasts and bodybuilders alike. It derives its popularity from its simplicity. Many, many offshoot programs can be accommodated within the general confines of the set system, and often are. The simplicity of the set system is hard to match. All that is required is that you exercise for the appropriate reps and sets, rest appropriately between sets, and then move on to the next exercise, continuing this until the end of the workout. It is not adaptable to cardiovascular training, generally, since rest periods are frequent. It is, however, the best system for improving limit strength, owing to the ample rest intervals. For review:

"Reps" is the abbreviation for repetitions. Repetitions define the number of times an exercise is to be performed. For example if you do 10 one-armed dumbbell rows and then stop, the 10 rows are considered 10 reps.

Performing a repetition or a group of repetitions and then stopping is a set. After performing 10 rows then stopping, doing that exercise again in the same training session would be a second set regardless of sequence; stop and start again would be a third set and so on.

Set System: Example Training Routine
- Lunge Squats (Rest 1-2 Minutes)
- Lunge Squats (Rest 1-2 Minutes)
- Lunge Squats (Rest 1-2 Minutes)
- Dumbbell Bench Press (Rest 1-2 Minutes)
- Dumbbell Bench Press (Rest 1-2 Minutes)
- Dumbbell Bench Press (Rest 1-2 Minutes)
  ...and so forth through workout

The Superset System/Complex Training

Supersetting (A "super set" is a very big set) is a term often used to describe alternating two exercises for the same body part (more appropriately referred to as "giant sets"), or alternating two exercises for different body parts (more appropriately referred to as "compound sets"). The traditional description of supersetting is that two anatomically antagonistic movements are alternately performed, and each movement is repeated alternately for the required number of reps; in the literature they are calling this "complex training for uniformity," we will stick with that term when referencing agonist/antagonist paired supersets.

For example, bench presses are supersetted with bent rows in the example below.

There is no rest between the two exercises comprising each super set. Do all repetitions back-to-back. Below is an example of a full superset workout. Between each superset, take a brief rest, just enough to allow the heart rate to fall back to a manageable level (approximately 100-120 beats per minute). Then go on to the next superset.

Superset	Exercises	Muscles Involved	Sequence
1	Dumbbell Bench Press Dumbbell Bent Rows (Elbows Out)	Pectorals Rhomboids	1 2 1 2 1 2 1 2
2	Crunches Dumbbell Back Raises	Abdominals Erector Spinae	3 4 3 4 3 4 3 4
3	Seated Dumbbell Presses One-Arm Dumbbell Bent Rows (Elbow Close to Side)	Deltoids Latissimus	5 6 5 6 5 6 5 6
4	Side Bends Left Side Bends Right	Internal And External Obliques	7 8 7 8 7 8 7 8
5	French Presses Dumbbell Biceps Curls	Triceps Biceps	9 10 9 10 9 10
6	Keystone Deadlifts Lunge Squats	Hamstrings Quadriceps	11 12 11 12 11 12 11 12

Science Speaks

A 2009 study published in the *Journal of Sports Sciences* entitled "Effects of agonist-antagonist complex resistance training on upper body strength and power development" demonstrated the efficiency of complex training. Over the course of eight weeks, a group that trained the bench press with bench pulls (an opposing pulling movement for the upper back) did improve bench press strength slightly over a group that trained the bench press with traditional sets.

While the complex training group did not have a statistically significant surge in bench press strength over the control group, the study did demonstrate the efficiency of complex training: the same amount of work could basically be done in half the time without compromising strength gains. This demonstrates that complex training is an effective means of cutting down time in the gym and continually making gains.

A 2005 study published in the *Journal of Strength and Conditioning Research* entitled "Acute effect on power output of alternating an agonist and antagonist muscle exercise during complex training" suggested that not only does complex training save time, but it potentially enhances power. The study found that rugby players with strength training experience increased power by 4.7 percent when training the bench press throw in a complex, as opposed to doing the bench press throw alone. Science says we will save time and not sacrifice strength and power gains from workouts and, quite possibly, even enhance them.

The Lab Meets the Real World

It is important to note that most advanced strength athletes do not train this way. The subjects in the aforementioned studies were not competitive lifters. We believe this is because of fatigue. Strength is a product of the Central Nervous System (CNS). Elite strength athletes have very efficient motor recruitment patterns. So, in lay terms, they are so skilled at the movements they perform that they fatigue faster. Studies have shown the stronger an individual is, the longer rest intervals need to be between sets. Remember, we are talking about elite strength athletes, not the vast majority of experienced gym lifters.

If this is you, there are a couple of ways you can handle this. Continue training with straight sets; the strongest men in the world have done this for centuries. The second option is what I call modified complex training (MCT). MCT simply means you pair an agonist and antagonist together like complex training.

But here's the kicker! Emphasize one of the movements. If you are capable of doing dumbbell overhead presses (OHP) 200 pounds and a pull-up with 80 pounds over your bodyweight for eight reps, emphasizing shoulders might look like this with MCT:

Set 1 MCT

OHP 170 Pounds × 5 Reps—Pull-ups Bodyweight × 5 reps

Set 2 MCT

OHP 170 Pounds × 4 Reps—Pull-ups Bodyweight × 5 reps

Set 3 MCT

OHP 170 Pounds × 3 Reps—Pull-ups Bodyweight × 5 reps

The inverse of MCT placing the emphasis on the upper back would look like this

Set 1 MCT

Pull-Up 80 Pounds Over Bodyweight × 8 Reps—OHP 110x8

Set 2 MCT

Pull-Up 80 Pounds Over Bodyweight × 6 Reps—OHP 110x8

Set 3 MCT

Pull-Up 80 Pounds Over Bodyweight × 5 Reps—OHP 110x8

This still allows extra stimulation of the antagonist muscle group without annihilating it.

Complex training is the ultimate method to increase training density. If time is of the essence, or if you just are looking to try something new, give complex training a shot!

Furthermore, antagonistic exercises alternating back and forth in the manner described will do two things. First, it will ensure that the blood supply is confined to a relatively small anatomical area, rather than having to alternately traverse the length of the body. This facilitates speedy recovery of the protagonist while the antagonist is working, and vice versa.

Second, by exercising the muscles on both sides of the joint(s), normal flexibility will be maintained, owing to a balance in the resting strength (muscle tone) between each.

hen exercising the entire body, each superset should progress to an area of the body far removed from the previous superset. This is to ensure that some of the same muscles aren't being used in back-to-back supersets, thereby preventing undue fatigue.

The Peripheral Heart Action Training System

Peripheral Heart Action Training (PHA) is circuit training on steroids! This was a favorite cutting strategy of bodybuilders in the 1960s. We are not talking pink dumbbells or the circuit training at your local Curves. Famous English philosopher, Thomas Hobbes, would describe PHA training as "nasty, brutish and short."

Sitting down is easier than standing up; that's why most circuit training stations consist of machines where you sit. Believe me, this is not about results, safety or efficiency. Simply, this is the path of the least resistance but also the path of the least results!

Burning calories may be your only goal but I don't think anyone would argue that a lot more calories are burned using compound movements with free weights standing up that allow for free movement, require force produced across multiple joints and require stability. This is harder and has a much higher metabolic cost during the workout and post workout.

Let's take a look at a system that does what circuit training hopes to do when it grows up.

PHA History

This system of bodybuilding circuit training was popularized to the masses by Bob Gajda, a Mr. Universe and Mr. America winner in the 1960s, but it was actually the brainchild of Chuck Coker, the inventor of the Universal Machine and mentor to cult bodybuilding legend, Chuck Sipes.

The idea is to keep blood circulating through the body throughout the entire workout, which is done by attacking the smaller muscles around the heart first, then moving outward. This system is vigorous and requires continued intense exercise for a prolonged period of time without any rest. Because of this, the poorly conditioned bodybuilder and the faint of heart will not do well with this training system.

The idea is to use primarily compound movements for efficiency. The goal is to "shunt" blood up and down the body; this is extremely taxing on the cardiovascular system, but the obvious benefits are a reduction in body fat and, of course, improved metabolic rate.

Because each sequential body part covered in each sequence is getting adequate rest between each circuit, strength will be conserved, allowing close to maximal strength to be exhibited on the sequential bout. Even though your heart will likely beat at over 150 beats per minute throughout the entire workout, this does not give you a license to lower weights; if you have the testicular fortitude, you should still be able to lift heavy on the rested body part.

Here is a PHA Circuit:

Sequence 1

- Dumbbell Overhead Press—8-10 reps

- Leg Raises—10-15 reps

- Pull-ups—8-10 reps

- Dumbbell Deadlifts—10-12 reps

- Repeat this sequence three times.

Sequence 2

- Weighted Dips—8-10 reps

- Dumbbell Bent Over Rows-8-10 reps

- Dumbbell Front Squats—6-8 reps

- Dumbbell French Press—10-12 reps

- Zottman Curls—10-12 reps

- Repeat this sequence three times.

*Perform the exercises in Sequence 1 for the required number of reps sequentially and do not stop! Repeat the sequence twice more, then move on to Sequence 2, performing it the same way you performed Sequence 1.

Do not rest during a sequence and do not rest between sequences unless absolutely necessary; after all, long breaks defeat the purpose. Maintain your heart rate at 80 percent of your heart rate max; wear a monitor so you can adjust the pace accordingly. If you are in shape, you will not have to trade heavy weight for a slower pace or longer rest.

Variable Manipulation

Your body is pretty smart, if you train the same way over and over, your body will adapt pretty quickly. With PHA training, to make progress, you have to continually overload. A variety of parameters can be manipulated to induce overload: increase the numbers of reps you have done with the same weight previously, increase the number of sequences, add weight on the bar, add chains, or increase frequency. The possibilities are endless. You will need to use a variety of rep ranges and training weight intensities.

Limit Strength

PHA training uses compound core exercises, so unlike machine circuit training, strength is your base regardless of endeavor. It is not the sacrificial lamb!

Free weight compound exercises are the most energy-demanding movements in the weight room. These are simply multi-joint movements that necessitate several different muscle groups to work together to the lift the weight; examples are pull-ups, overhead presses, dips, squats, deadlifts and bench presses. These movements burn more fuel because they involve more muscles and allow heavier weights to be used. Try a maximum intensity set of 20 dumbbell deadlifts, and then do the same intensity with 20 cable bicep curls; it should be obvious that you expend a lot more energy with the dumbbell deadlifts.

Compound movements catalyze a cascade release of the good hormones like testosterone and growth hormone naturally, which facilitates muscle growth and fat loss. Whether bulking up or cutting down, compound movements are the "base" of your training. Compound movements need to be the mainstay of PHA training. As long as you are in good shape, you still have to train heavy!

PHA training has fallen out of favor with many mainstream fitness authorities and celebrity personal trainers. Client retention would be miniscule for "general fitness" trainees with such a demanding methodology. But before illegal anabolic drugs hi-jacked many sound training principles and systems, PHA training helped construct many championship-caliber, lean and muscular physiques. If you are looking for something new, want a challenge and are pressed for time, give PHA training a shot.

The below PHA sequence, designed by Fred Hatfield, caught on like wild fire in the 1990s.

The Peripheral Heart Action Training System

Exercise Sequence 1

- Dumbbell Partial Press
- Crunches
- Lunge Squats
- French Presses

Exercise Sequence 2

- Forearm Curls
- One-Arm Dumbbell Rows (elbow close to side)
- Dumbbell Back Raises
- Dips
- Bicep Curls

Exercise Sequence 3

- Reverse Forearm Curls
- Side Bends
- Leg Extensions
- Keystone Deadlifts

Exercise Sequence 4

- Dumbbell Bench Presses
- Bent Rows (elbows out)
- Shrugs
- Forearm Supinations (Thor's Hammer)

Performance

Perform the exercises in Sequence 1 for the required number of reps, working nonstop. Repeat the sequence two more times, and progress on to Sequence 2, performing this sequence three times as well. Then, progress through Sequence 3 and Sequence 4 in the same fashion. Go nonstop throughout, except when your heart rate exceeds the required 140-160 beats per minute, in which case, either slow down or rest briefly.

The principle functions of the PHA system are to increase cardiovascular efficiency; to maintain flexibility (S1 is "supersetted" with S2, and S3 with S4); to increase strength and size in synergists, stabilizers and prime movers; and, in an encapsulating effect, to afford you with a sound foundation of overall fitness. The key is to make the reps of each set rhythmic, with a brief (1-2 seconds) rest pause between each rep. This will reduce the "pressor response" usually inherent in weight training, which tends to negate cardiovascular benefit.

Notice that the exercises in each sequence are chosen on the basis of how far removed one is from the other. The exercises traverse your entire body in each sequence, forcing blood to be shunted up and down your body. This will offer cardiovascular benefits, but also allow recovery of each area before "blitzing" it again. For while the heart is working hard, the refreshed muscle can endure maximal overload again and again, due to the long periods of active rest between each exercise.

Circuit Training System

Circuit training, "the little brother of PHA training," is still an excellent system for beginners aspiring to improve general fitness. The main objective in completing all of the stations in the circuit is decreased time. You should choose the exercises most important to your sport or those exercises most important from the standpoint of eliminating your weaknesses. The most important exercises are placed early in the circuit and the least important ones later in the circuit. You then perform each exercise in succession, attempting always to better your "target time." The main objective is density; instead of blindly tacking exercises you have to continually strive to do the same amount of volume in less time. The idea is that cardiovascular efficiency and increased strength and tonus will result. As target times are achieved, or as new weaknesses crop up, you should change the circuit accordingly.

Example Circuit

1. Lunge Squats
2. Dumbbell Bent Rows
3. Curls
4. Clean Pulls
5. Dumbbell Bench Press
6. Triceps Kickbacks
7. Crunches
8. Overhead Dumbbell Presses

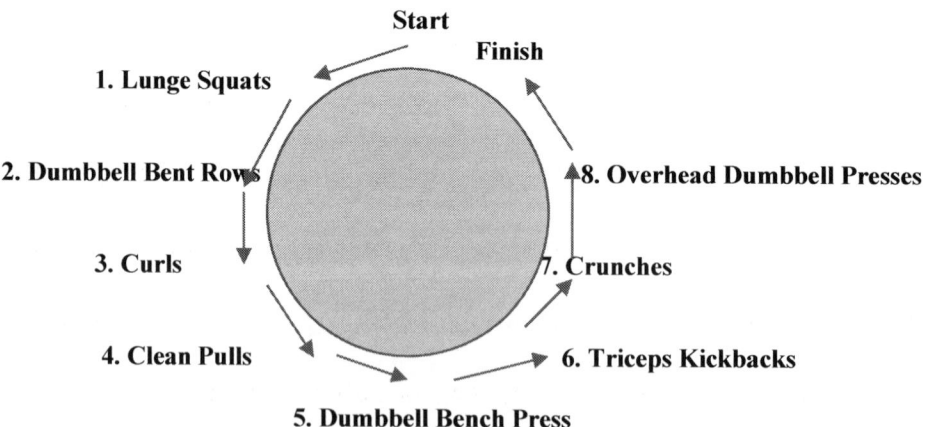

The circuit may be repeated for as many sets as desired, either by resting between sets at each station or by going through the circuit non-stop several times.

Naturally, the amount of resistance used at each station will vary depending on individual differences in strength and stamina. Make the reps of each set rhythmic, with a brief (1-2 seconds) rest pause between each. This will reduce the "pressor response" usually inherent in weight training, which tends to negate cardiovascular benefit.

Notice also that each station in sequence tends to involve body areas far removed from each other, a practice designed to avoid undue fatigue in any given muscle or muscle group, hampering your efforts to derive maximum overload.

Achieving elite-levels of limit strength or aerobic conditioning will not happen with circuit training. However, both objectives can get more possible very quickly for the untrained individual or general fitness enthusiast.

Mixed Systems

Remember, these systems are not put in here to play follow the leader; they are simply guidelines to help you develop the optimal training program. Many of the systems presented can be mixed, depending on training objective. You can also easily incorporate one system into another, as was the case with "supersetting" in the PHA System.

As you get to know your limitations and idiosyncrasies with respect to how you respond to these systems, you'll see what works best for one aspect of fitness may not be so effective for another. Different body parts may respond better or worse to the different systems. By the time you have trained for about a year—less for some—you will have picked out those systems that best serve your needs and may decide to mix systems. This is our goal for you!

As one progresses toward training goals, you might outgrow a system. That is, as a muscle develops and adapts to the challenge you have imposed upon it, you may be obliged to change systems in order to force continued development—do not allow progress to wane.

Remember to have fun!

Extreme Strength and Hypertrophy Methods

Some of you are advanced bodybuilders and need extreme methods to push past strength and muscle-building stalemates. The following methods offer a high reward, but they also carry a higher risk. These methods should be reserved for injury-free, advanced trainees with at least two years of consistent weight training experience.

Compensatory Acceleration Training

Two people can do the exact same workout program, but one gets superior results! No, it is not because of genetics. The secret lies in performance of the reps during training. One gets maximum overload each set, each rep and each workout. The superior lifter does this 100 percent of the time, while most trainees are lucky to do the same 20 percent of the time.

Movement Intention

If you wish to move big weights, you need to have the intention of moving the dumbbells as fast as possible on compound movements. We call this "movement intention." Lifting lighter weights fast provides many of the benefits of training heavy. Unsurprisingly, lifting heavy weights with intent to move them fast builds explosive strength. Ultimately, your body will adapt to the intent of your CNS to move weight explosively.

Improving Leverage

Performing dumbbell bench presses is the most demanding at the bottom of the rep. So many gym rats believe that once they reach the half-way point, they can cash in on the improvement in leverage and positional strength to coast through the rep until lockout. Wrong!

With improved leverage at the half-way position you want to *compensate* by moving the weight faster—this is Compensatory Acceleration Training (CAT). The overriding training benefit of CAT is that it forces your muscles to produce maximal force through the entire range of motion. Think this sounds dangerous? As published in the International Sports Science Association (ISSA) personal training certification many decades ago, "Slamming a weight to the end point in the range of motion certainly would cause injury. The 'learning curve' involved in slowing the movement down just before lockout is very small. Anyone can learn how to do it on the first try."

Example

For your next workout, say that you are dumbbell bench pressing four sets of five reps, using the same weight each set. Most folks start each rep explosive out of the bottom, but coast to the finish.

Here is a typical scenario.

> **Set 1**—No dumbbell bench presses were heavy enough to stimulate any overload. That is a zero percent efficiency rating.

> **Set 2**—The bottom half of the last rep required enough intensity for overload, which is a 10 percent efficiency rating.

> **Set 3**—The bottom half of the last two reps provided overload, and that is a 20 percent efficiency rating.

> **Set 4**—The bottom half of all five reps produced overload. That is two and a half, still a 50 percent efficiency rating.

The workout was 20 total repetitions; only eight halves produced overload or helped you get stronger. This equates to a 20 percent efficiency rating. That sucks! Try telling your boss that you're 20 percent efficient and you'll be in line at the soup kitchen.

Over weeks, months and years, two people on the exact same program will get totally different results. One is a physical specimen, the other is cannon fodder!

If all 20 reps were pressed with maximal force, you'd be much stronger over time. Force equals mass × x acceleration. Lifting lighter weights in CAT style enables you to produce maximal force with less strain on your central nervous system.

The slow and controlled dogma has haunted the fitness establishment for decades. Next time the personal trainer at the "chrome palace gym" puts down his soy latte to make doctrinal claims about gaining strength, call his bluff and tell him to take his "bro science" to a more gullible audience.

Bottom line—size and strength is gained by training core lifts in a CAT style.

Rest-Pause Training

With "three hots and a cot," recovery time and all the pig iron one could handle on the jailhouse weight pile, Jim Williams (a.k.a. "The Scranton Strongman") resided behind prison walls. While serving time for a string of youthful indiscretions, Williams turned his jail sentence into an opportunity to experiment with new iron game ideas and transformed himself into the prison's strongest inmate. His weight lifting innovations paid enormous dividends, as illustrated when he became the first person to surpass a 650 pound bench press in competition. Williams wasn't a one trick pony. He totaled an astounding 2,240 pounds in a full meet following time served. Prisons don't boast state of the art equipment or people with Ph.D.s in exercise physiology running around to ensure that cons train in accordance with the latest lab study. What prisons do offer is a significant amount of time for inmates to exchange physical culture knowledge and to develop their own strategies for getting bigger and stronger.

Jim Williams never had a world-class strength coach; he wore prison-issued denim instead of spandex and didn't have access to bands or chains. Nevertheless, he was able to develop legendary strength and size via the rest-pause method.

According to numerous interviews Adam benShea and Josh Bryant conducted for their best-selling book, *Jailhouse Strong*, prison bodybuilding legends Michael Christian and Tookie Williams trained with a high-rep variation of the rest-pause method.

So, why did the rest-pause method evolve out of the jailhouse weight pile? The answer is simple: With limited weights on the yard, you can't give up your spot on the bench press.

Hence, do as many reps as possible ... take a short break ... repeat.

Once again, we see that necessity is the mother of invention!

Rest-Pause Training Explained

Rest-pause training breaks down one set into several sub-sets with a brief rest between each. Depending on the intensity level and training objectives, several different variations may be used.

If strength is your priority, take a note from the "Scranton Strongman." Williams took 90 to 95 percent of his one-repetition max, waited 20 to 60 seconds and then performed another single. He repeated the process for the maximum amount of sets that he could do that day. Typically, he did six to eight singles. This method is extremely taxing on the central nervous system. So, proceed with caution! The training adaptations with this variation are more neurologically driven for strength, rather than muscle size.

Doing heavy singles with a dumbbell is not practical but we can take a play out of Michael Christian's playbook.

If hypertrophy is what you're after, lighten the load but maintain the training intensity. Select your chosen dumbbell exercise and load a weight that you can perform for six to 10 repetitions. Lift the weight for as many reps as possible, take a 20-second rest interval, and do the same weight again. This next set will probably be two to three repetitions. Repeat this process twice, for a total of three sub sets.

Why It Works

Each lifter has differences that eventually dictate how many reps and sets he can perform, how often he can train, and how much weight he should be using while training. The nature of rest-pause training allows it to be custom tailored to individual differences! Regardless of one's ability to perform reps, maximum intensity is the ingredient that induces size and strength gains.

Fast Gainer/Slow Gainer Rep Ranges

To completely develop the physique you're looking for, you must take a holistic approach to training. In other words, volume, tempo, reps and sets must vary. For the most part, fast gainers will experience their best gains with lower reps and slow gainers with higher reps.

The five sets of five repetitions strength program with 85 percent of a lifter's one-rep max would be extremely difficult for a fast gainer, yet impossible for some. For a slow gainer, this would be moderate intensity and provide very little adaptive overload.

A rest-pause set on the dumbbell bench press for a true fast gainer with 85 percent of his one-repetition max could look something like this: 85 percent × 3 reps, rest 30 seconds, 85 percent × 1 rep, rest 30 seconds, 85 percent × 1 rep. Bottom line is the fast gainer performed five repetitions over three mini sets; that's the most he can. Since fast gainers make their greatest gains with low reps, he will get bigger and stronger.

The true slow gainer with the same weight over three mini sets with identical rest intervals may have performed a sequence that went 13 reps, seven reps and five reps; that is a total of 25 reps. Since that is maximum intensity and the slow gainer thrives on high reps, he will get bigger and stronger.

Unlike traditional single-repetition rest pauses that old-time strength athletes swear by, open ended rest-pause training (i.e. doing as many reps as possible each mini set) allows the athlete to adapt the weight to his individual capabilities. A primarily slow-twitch lifter will get more reps; a fast-twitch lifter will get fewer reps. Both experience an adaptive overload since maximal intensity is tailored to their individual differences.

Bottom line is both the slow gainer and fast gainer are performing their sets with an all-out effort; maximum intensity tailored to individual genetic make-up is synergy for great results. Here is an example of a rest-pause dumbbell bench press workout.

Rest-Pause Dumbbell Bench Press workout:

- Set 1—80 percent As Many As Possible (AMAP), rest 20-30 seconds 80 percent AMAP, rest 20-30 seconds 80 percent AMAP

- Rest 2-5 minutes

- Set 2—70 percent AMAP, rest 20-30 seconds 70 percent AMAP, rest 20-30 seconds 70 percent AMAP

Rest-pausing is taxing on the central nervous system (CNS) and should not be used every workout, or every set. Also, avoid using this method for highly technical movements (i.e., Olympic lifting variations).

Nonetheless, under the right tutelage, rest-pause training can offer some amazing results. Fortunately, you do not have to be a jailhouse denizen to try it. So give it a shot!

Time Under Tension Training

This ain't your daddy's "Super Slow Training!"

Get through the set. Get through the set. Get through the set. This is usually what runs through your mind when trying to hit a target number of reps. The problem, however, is that you become more concerned with reaching rep 10 than with crushing reps one through nine. If you're concerned at all with muscle growth, this is a bad practice. By simply "getting through" the set, you're failing to take advantage of all the benefits each rep has to offer.

Make Use of Time

To slow things down—while speeding up growth—try taking stock of your total muscular time under tension. Reps will still count but now they will count for a lot more. Read on to learn how to make time under tension, or TUT, work for you.

Research

Scientists have hypothesized that muscle hypertrophy is not purely a function of rep ranges but the actual duration of the set. One recent study from McMaster University in Canada published in the *Journal of Physiology* seemed to confirm that prolonged muscle contraction was the most important variable for increasing muscle size. The study compared light loads using a tempo of one second up and one second down or using slow reps of six seconds up and six seconds down. The study found the slow reps were superior because of the amount of time that working muscles were under tension.

However, the findings of armchair academics and lab geeks must be interpreted with a grain of salt. Studies can have flaws, typically because they are performed on malnourished, sleep-

68

deprived, hard-partying college kids looking for research dough, not the old heads that have been slinging iron in the trenches for years.

The aforementioned study compared explosive repetitions and slow repetitions with 30 percent of the subject's one-rep max. No one serious about getting stronger or packing on as much muscle as possible is doing 30 percent of their one-rep max for serious work sets. To put it in perspective, that would mean if you bench press 200 pounds, you would workout with 60 pounds with a goal of packing on serious muscle.

TUT is King

So what's the right approach when it comes to time under tension? We favor looking at it in the full context of growth-influencing factors.

Mechanical tension is related to exercise intensity (the amount of weight you are lifting). In other words, to get big you have to train heavy. Eight-time Mr. Olympia, Lee Haney, once said, "The key to building massive, powerful muscles is to doggedly increase the training weights you use." Science backs Haney, as does anecdotal evidence. I am not going to argue with Mr. Haney—neither should you.

Muscle damage is associated with muscle soreness; this inflammatory response aids in the muscle-building process, of course, assuming the lifter recovers properly.

Metabolic stress is a result of the byproducts of anaerobic metabolism in the 30- to 60-second range of set duration. In other words, lifting all-out for this duration of time, scientists believe, causes a huge spike in the anabolic hormones—growth hormone and IGF-1 (insulin-like growth factor). Adding icing to the cake, metabolic stress increases excess post-exercise oxygen consumption or EPOC, allowing you to burn more calories at rest and expediting fat loss.

The previously mentioned study isn't a total farce. However, it only sheds light on metabolic stress. To get the full beef-building payoff, you have to utilize time under tension training, with a close eye on mechanical tension, muscle damage and metabolic stress. The following workout gives you the chance to do all of that.

The Workouts

Chest and Back TUT Workout

> Superset I   Dumbbell Incline Press—Neutral-Grip Pull-Up

> Superset II   Dip--Dumbbell Pull Over

> Superset III   Dumbbell Fly—One-Arm Dumbbell Row

Leg and Bicep TUT Workout

> Superset I   Dumbbell Squats—Incline Dumbbell Curl

> Superset II   Dumbbell Keystone Deadlift—Keystone Deadlifts

> Superset III   Bodyweight Squats—Zottman Curls

Shoulders and Triceps TUT Workout

> Superset I   Dumbbell Military Press—Dumbbell Reverse Fly

> Superset II   Dumbbell Incline Lateral Raise—Decline Dumbbell Triceps Extensions

> Superset III   Dumbbell Front Raises—Lying Dumbbell Triceps Extension

Perform the first exercise listed for 30 seconds then begin the second one immediately and go for another 30 seconds. Take a two-minute rest after each superset.

TUT Exploits Hypertrophy Mechanisms

Muscle hypertrophy is a product of muscle damage, mechanical tension and metabolic stress. The time under tension method, done with maximum intensity, exploits all three hypertrophic mechanisms. Remember, keep on moving the entire time—even an eighth of an inch qualifies! Time under tension is one more weapon at your disposal in the muscle-building war.

TUT Guidelines

1. Control the negative reps (2-3 second negative) and explode on positives.

2. The goal is to keep the weight moving; if you reach momentary muscular failure (MMF) continue with partials. DO NOT DROP THE WEIGHT!! One millimeter is movement.

3. Start with weights you can do for a true rep max of 8-12 reps, shoot for 10-15 including partial contractions.

4. On each set, reduce load by approximately 1/3, so if you start with 90 pounds, set two would be with 60 pounds and set three with 40 pounds.

5. This technique is very high intensity. Do it for a maximum of three to four weeks before taking a light deload week.

6. Weekly progression can add 5-10 seconds per set, keeping the rest interval the same or keeping the time constant but increasing weight.

7. Use primarily bilateral movements with dumbbells (ones that use two limbs), i.e. both limbs contracting simultaneously. There are exceptions to this rule; it is majority of the time not all the time.

Final Thoughts

There are a plethora of high-intensity techniques for the advanced bodybuilder: traditional drop sets, rack and run, forced reps and a host of others. Instead of haphazardly offering a couple sentences about every possible technique, we wanted to share the ones we have used most effectively with clients and offer detailed explanations. Additionally, these are methods that can be done by those that train alone. These techniques are highly intense and highly effective. But anytime anything is taken to the extreme, the inherent risk involved increases.

Chapter VIII: Dumbbell Training Guidelines

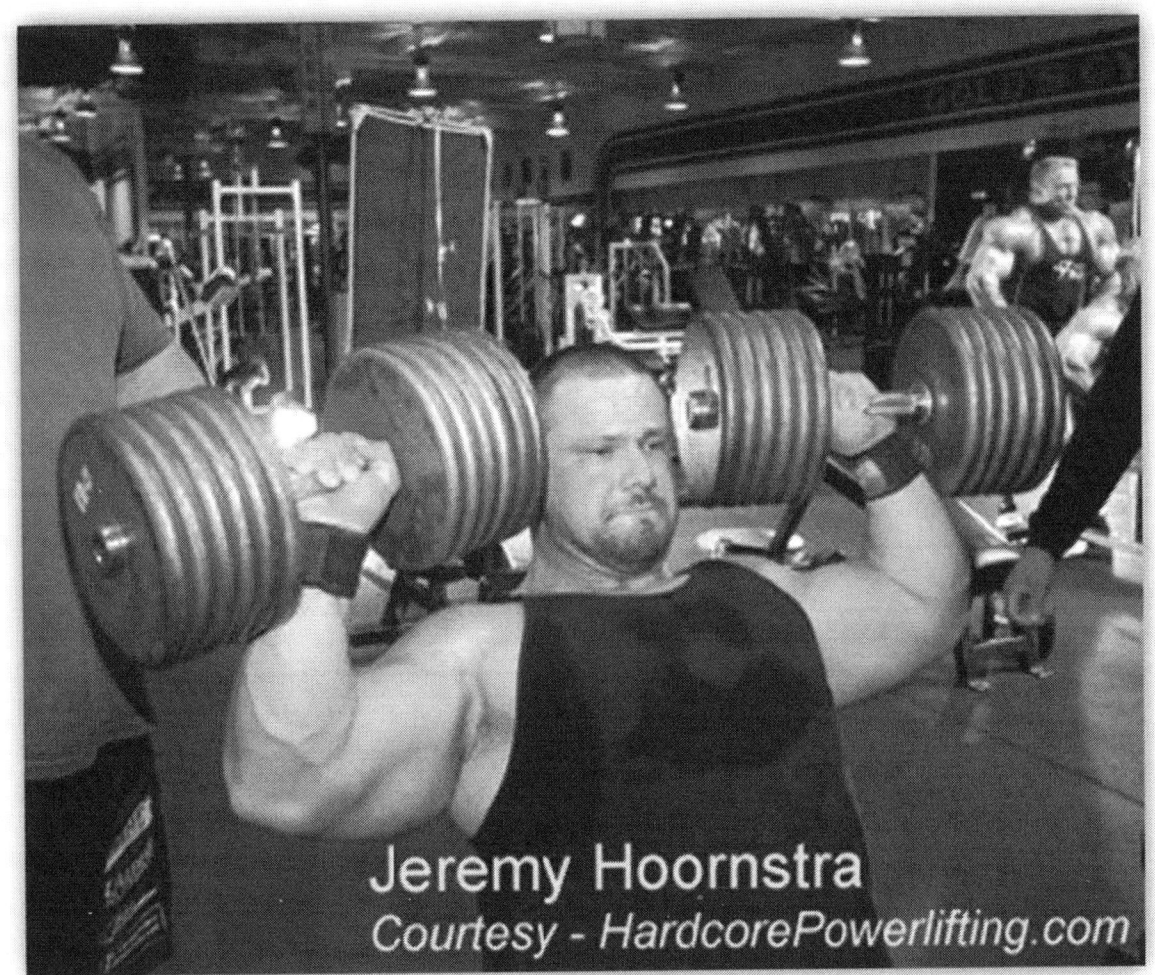

Jeremy Hoornstra
Courtesy - HardcorePowerlifting.com

For some of you, this may serve as a review but still read it. Following these basic guidelines decreases the chance of injury and increases the probability of your desired outcome.

Weight

Before starting an exercise, be sure that you have a feel for the exercise. Never "load up" an exercise with which you are unfamiliar or while in an extended body position. Increasing the resistance should always be done, but *after* you have a thoroughly comfortable feel for the exercise movement.

Machines

While this is a dumbbell training manual, we offer some advice when training with machines. We offer this word of caution.

If you are unfamiliar with how the machine you are about to use can be adjusted to your body, check with the certified trainer working at the gym. So many new models of gym equipment are on the market nowadays that you can't know the ins and outs of how to use all of them. Always make certain that all your equipment works properly before using it.

Breathing

Two general rules about breathing should be followed when working out:

1. Do not hold your breath continuously for several consecutive repetitions.

2. Try to develop a rhythmic pattern of breathing that corresponds to the exercise cycle. Exhale during the most strenuous (concentric) portion of each repetition and inhale during the least strenuous (eccentric) portion.

Holding your breath during an entire set of repetitions can lead to dizziness and possible fainting, among other more serious complications. Here is an example of proper breathing during a military (overhead) press repetition: Inhale as you bring the dumbbells toward your shoulders during the eccentric phase of the repetition. Exhale as your arms extend upward over your head. Exhale slowly and continuously. When you finish the press, you should have no more air in your lungs and should be ready to inhale for the eccentric (down) phase. For advanced lifters using large amounts of weight on compound movements like rows, pulls, presses, squats or any other multi-joint movement, we recommend the Valsalva maneuver.

How to perform the Valsalva maneuver:

1. Inhale before or during the negative. Once inhalation is complete, hold your breath and complete the negative.

2. Exhale against closed glottis at start of the positive. The positive starts by exhaling against the closed glottis (structure in windpipe, prevents air from passing if closed, allows passage of air when open). Your abs should be braced tight.

3. Exhale after sticking point and complete the positive. You are not holding your breath until you pass out. Once you pass the sticking point or complete the repetition, you can breathe.

4. Repeat the process for the remaining repetitions in your set.

Why the Valsalva Maneuver?

Increased intra-abdominal and intra-thoracic pressure reduces the load on the lower and middle back and effectively enhances both of these areas' ability to transmit force.

Studies have shown higher force production capabilities with the Valsalva maneuver. The middle-aged businessman with high blood pressure looking to get healthy is advised against this technique. Consideration is for the serious physique or strength enthusiast.

Outcries against the Valsalva maneuver are speculative bro science.

Warm-ups

People tend to take warming up for granted. Pump a few weights, jog in place, and WHAM! Hit the heavy stuff. Well, it's not that simple.

The theoretical purposes of warm-up exercises include:

1. increased muscle temperature associated with enhanced dissociation of oxygen from red blood cells,

2. improved metabolic adjustment to heavy work,

3. increased velocity of nerve conduction,

4. greater numbers of capillaries opened in the muscles, and

5. several psychological factors.

Skilled performances improve with warm-ups using activity identical or directly related to the sport. Prior physical activity improves the "mental set" or attitude of the athlete, especially when the activity is identical or directly related to the skill. Warm-ups cause an increased "arousal," or enthusiasm, eagerness and mental readiness. But there is one potentially negative effect of warm-ups—fatigue from the prior activity can decrease performance.

Most people who work out have accepted the need to warm up as dogma. Clinically, there appears to be some support for warming up as a deterrent to injury, but it certainly doesn't apply in all cases. For example:

1. Athletes engaged in short, explosive types of sports such as powerlifting benefit from warming up for improved performance.

2. Athletes engaged in progressive-type sports or endurance events do not benefit from warming up.

3. Warming up before an endurance-type sport often will decrease performance because of fatigue.

4. Direct warm-ups (exercise directly related or the same as the sport) of moderate intensity and duration prior to explosive sports enhance trained athletes' performance, but not necessarily that of untrained athletes.

5. Indirect warm-ups (exercise not directly related to the sport) often can aid performance, as can bicycling for four to five minutes or flexibility (stretching) exercises.

6. Almost all studies showing a detrimental effect from warming up used untrained people as the subjects, who apparently cannot tolerate high-intensity warm-ups.

7. Heavy, unrelated warm-ups interfere with one's ability to perform sports skills requiring careful control.

8. Your warm-up should ensure improved performance, and only careful experimenting will yield the best type, intensity and duration for you.

Overview

In general, it seems that the widely held belief in warming up prior to training or competition needs to be carefully considered before a specific warm-up program is adopted.

In weight training, there appears to be little justification for warming up at any vigorous level. Typically, the exercise itself serves as sufficient warm-up. But unlike in other sports, there's probably no good reason *not* to warm up either. If you decide to use a mild warm-up, use lighter weights for the targeted muscles or a general warm-up until you're lightly sweating.

One final point on warm-ups: *Never* do flexibility exercises as a warm-up. Vigorously stretching a cold muscle is the easiest way to inflict microtrauma or (worse) macrotrauma—full-blown injury.

Generally one to two warm-up sets of the exercise will suffice, but some people need more. If this is you, try this dynamic stretching routine after a five-to-eight-minute warm-up.

We do recommend dynamic stretching prior to training. Dynamic stretching before your workout reduces the chance of injury and enhances proprioceptors, which allows you to produce more power and strength. Dynamic stretching should be performed after a 10-minute general warm-up such as a brisk walk or ride on an exercise bike.

Sample Dynamic Stretching Routine

- Walk on toes—2 sets 15 yards

- Arm Swings—2 sets of 10 clockwise and counterclockwise

- Arm Hugs—2 sets 10 reps

- Straight Leg Kicks—3 sets 15 yards

- Leg Swings—2 sets 15 reps

- High Knees—3 sets 15 yards

- Walking Lunges—3 sets 15 yards

- Butt Kicks—3 sets 15 yards

- Wrist Sways—3 sets 15 each way

- Twists in place—3 sets 15 each way

- Clockwise and counterclockwise hula hoop hip swings, 2 sets 10 both ways

Upon completing this warm-up, the athlete would start to move into lighter weights of the exercise of the upcoming routine at a gradually increasing pace.

Cool-Down

At the end of each exercise session, perform some cool-down movements for five or 10 minutes. This is especially important after high-intensity exercise, which contains an anaerobic component (for example, very high-resistance training such as bodybuilding).

Sample Cool-Down Program

Static Stretch (Do each stretch for 30 seconds)

- Pectoralis Stretch
- Latissimus Stretch
- Bicep Stretch
- Triceps Stretch
- Forearm Flexor Stretch
- Forearm Extensor Stretch
- Standing Quadriceps Stretch
- Psoas Stretch
- Rectus Femoris Stretch
- Adductor Stretch
- Sumo Squat Stretch
- Frog Stretch
- Erector Spinae Stretch
- Piriformis Stretch
- Hamstrings 90/90 Stretch
- Hamstring w/Adduction
- Gastrocnemius
- Soleus

Peroneal Stretch

- SFMR (Foam Rolling)
- Roll tender spots for 20 seconds, 1 set each spot
- Hamstrings and Calves
- Gluteus Medius
- IT Band/Tensor Fascia Latae
- Quadriceps/Hip Flexors
- Adductor
- Low-Back/Erector Spinae

- Rhomboids
- Latissimus Dorsi

Final Thoughts

The poorest way to recover is to simply fall to the ground or sit around!

The rhythmic contractions of your mildly active muscles help return blood to your heart. Many pints of blood are distributed, supplying needed oxygen and nutrients (especially glucose for replacement of spent energy from muscle glycogen, and amino acids for repair and growth). So give your heart some help with light aerobic cool-down activities.

The cool-down should also contain mild stretching exercises for the muscles you just finished training. This will assist in avoiding post-exercise muscle soreness by breaking up tiny adhesions resulting from the "microtrauma" they've just suffered during training. For all these reasons, it'll also assist your working muscles during exercise, and will tend to pool there, rather than aiding in swift removal of wastes and affected muscles' recovery.

Remember, Rome was not built in a day; follow these guidelines to optimize gains and minimize risks.

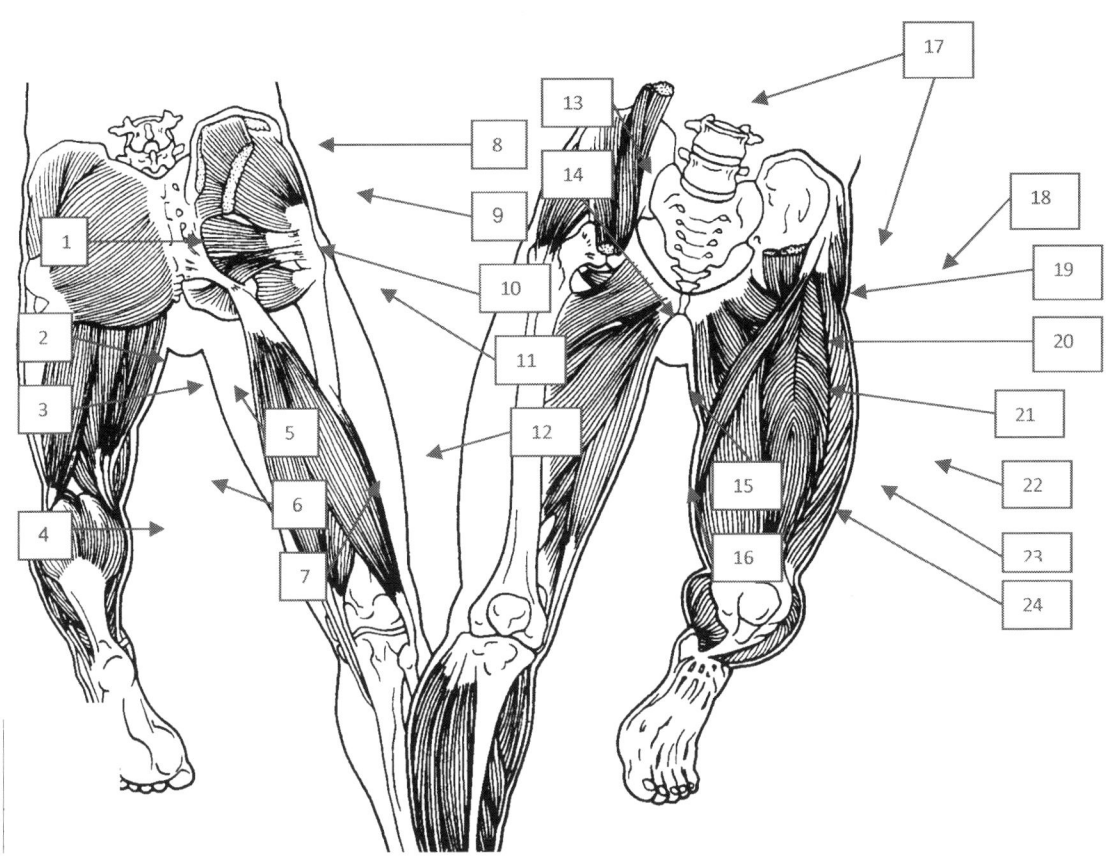

1. Gleuteus Maximus	13. Tensor Fascia Latae
2. Biceps Femoris	14. Pectineus
3. Semitendinosus	15. Adductor Longus
4. Gastrocnemius	16. Adductor Magnus
5. Gracilis	17. Iliopsoas (Sectioned)
6. Semimembranosus	18. Tensor Fascia Latae
7. Semimembranosus	19. Pectineus
8. Glutcus Medius	20. Adductor Longus
9. Gluteus Minimus	21. Sartorius
10. Piriformis	22. Vastus Lateralis
11. Quadratus Femoris	23. Rectus Femoris
12. Biceps Femoris	24. Vastus Lateralis

Nothing looks as silly as the bodybuilder with a massive upper body and a massively under-

developed lower body!

Leg development, while important to aesthetics, is paramount for athletic success in anything from schoolyard scuffles to lawn bowling; very powerful legs can be developed with dumbbells.

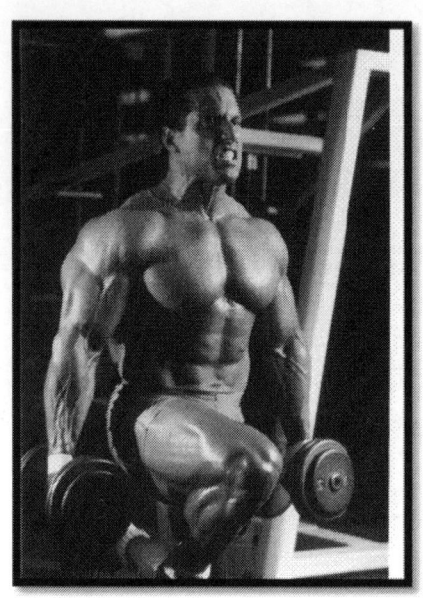

While there are methods of isolating the individual muscles of your legs and hips, my experience tells me that functional strength and sports performance abilities are more effectively developed using compound exercises. That is, exercises that require all of the muscles of your upper legs and hips to work synchronously.

There are many great leg exercises; let's take a look at a few of our favorites.

Dumbbell Lunges

With front lunges, you're actually simulating a one-legged squat.

Exercise Performance

1. Stand with your torso upright holding two dumbbells at your sides. This is the starting position.

2. Step forward with your right leg around two feet or so from the foot being held stationary and lower your upper body down, while keeping the torso upright and maintaining balance. Do not allow your knee to go forward beyond your toes as you go down. Keep your front shin perpendicular to the ground. The dumbbells are now hanging alongside the forward leg instead of at your sides.

3. Using primarily the heel of your foot, push straight upward and go back to the starting position as you exhale. A common mistake is to lean forward as you "stride" forward

while ascending back to the starting position. This creates undue shear on the forward knee, and low back stress.

4. Repeat for the prescribed repetitions.

Important Notes:

Alternate legs going right, left, right then left. For advanced athletes, walking dumbbell lunges can be a viable option: Perform the same movement walking forward in a lunging pattern. Opt for a set distance like 15-20 yards; the goal is to accomplish this in as few steps as possible.

An Interesting Variation:

Instead of stepping directly forward with each rep, try stepping slightly left and right alternately. You can also move laterally, backward and forward while twisting left or right.

Step-Ups

Also called the "simulated mountain climb," step-ups are an offshoot of the old "Harvard Step Test." This test was originally designed to assess physical work capacity (PWC), and involved stepping up onto a bench 20 inches high for five minutes and at a cadence of 30 step-ups per minute.

Well, you can imagine how difficult this test would be for a shorter person! So let's forget the cadence and time limit and lower the height to a normal gym bench (usually 14-16 inches in height). If such a bench is still too high, you can perform this exercise using the shorter blocks typically used in aerobics classes (e.g., the Reebok steps).

Exercise Performance

1. Grab a pair of dumbbells and hold them down at your sides.

2. Stand up straight in front of a raised platform, facing straight ahead; this is the starting position.

3. Lift your left knee and step onto the platform with your left foot.

4. Firmly plant your foot on the platform, use your left heel to lift your body up and place your right foot on the platform as well. Important note: All of the force should be produced with the left leg; this is a single-leg movement. Also, you may find it more comfortable if you allow the dumbbells to hang alongside your forward leg instead of at your sides.

5. Briefly pause at the top of the movement and then step back with your right leg and safely return to the starting position.

6. Repeat prescribed repetitions.

Important Notes:

Never allow your back to round. Keep your head up and back straight throughout the exercise. A higher platform is a more intense exercise. Think beyond just weight, sets, reps, rest intervals. Start by using just bodyweight. A great deal of balance is required and caution should be used.

Keystone Deadlifts

So-named because the position you assume resembles that of the old-time "Keystone Cops," with your butt and belly protruding (lower back is arched). This position causes your hamstrings (back of thigh) to become pre-stretched. Then, while keeping your back arched, lower the dumbbells alongside your legs until they reach your knees, and stand back up. It is an excellent exercise for the hamstrings.

Exercise Performance

1. Grasp two dumbbells, holding the weight in front of you.

2. Bend the knees slightly and keep the shins vertical, hips back and back straight. This will be your starting position.

3. Keeping your back and arms completely straight at all times, push your butt back and bend at the waist.

4. Lower the dumbbells by pushing the hips back, only slightly bending the knees; think a hinge not a squat. The dumbbells remain in contact with your thigh the entire movement.

5. Lower the dumbbells to just right below the knees.

6. Extend hips back to the starting point.

7. Repeat for prescribed number of repetitions.

Important Notes: Avoid this movement if you have lower back problems; avoid rounding of the back at all costs.

Bulgarian Split Squats

This movement hammers the quadriceps and glutes and provides some stimulation to the hamstrings and calves. More and more mainstream strength coaches are advocating the Bulgarian Split Squat.

Exercise Performance

Grab a pair of dumbbells and hold them at arm's length next to your sides.

1. Stand in a staggered stance, your left foot in front of your right. Set your feet two to three feet apart.

2. Place just the instep of your back foot on a bench. When you're doing split squats, the higher your foot is elevated, the harder the exercise.

3. Your front knee should be slightly bent.

4. Brace your core.

5. Begin the descent by flexing your knee and hip to lower your body down. Maintain a braced, upright posture the entire movement. Keep the front knee in line with the foot as you perform the exercise.

6. From the bottom of the movement, drive through the heel to extend the knee and hip to return to the starting position.

One-Leg Romanian Deadlift

This exercise is an old favorite of fabled sprints coach, the late Charlie Francis. This is one of the great hamstring exercises in existence and should be considered essential in the repertoire of any serious speed training athlete or, hell, anyone who wants some beautiful "strings of ham."

There was a reason why when Charlie Francis was at the helm of the Canadian Sprints program, injury rates of sprinters were comparable to those of distance runners.

Legendary sprinter Ben Johnson performed this movement with a pair of 150-pound dumbbells for six reps.

Exercise Performance

1. Hold a dumbbell in each hand. Position dumbbells down in front of upper thighs with arms straight. Stand with your feet together.

2. Lift one leg slightly so the foot is just off floor.

3. Keeping the core tight, lower the dumbbells to the floor while raising the lifted leg behind you.

4. Keep your back straight and the knee of the supporting leg slightly bent. Keep the hip and knee of lifted leg extended throughout movement.

5. Once a good stretch is felt or the dumbbells make contact with the floor, come back to the starting position. Repeat desired number of reps subsequently on the same leg or in an alternating fashion.

Dumbbell Squats

You Ain't Been Squattin
By Dale Clark 1983
Way Down the Road in a Gym Far Away
A Young Man Was Once Heard To Say
"I've Repped High and I've Repped Low"
"No Matter What I Do My Legs Won't Grow"
He Tried Leg Extension, Leg Curls and Leg Presses Too
Trying to Cheat These Sissy Workouts He'd Do
From The Corner of the Gym Where the Big Men Train
Through A Cloud of Chalk and the Midst of Pain
Where the Big Iron Rides High and Threatens Lives

Where the Noise Is Made With Big Forty Fives
A Deep Voice Bellowed As He Wrapped His Knees
A Very Big Man with Legs like Trees
Laughing As He Snatched another Plate from The Stack
Chalking His Hands and His Monstrous Back
Said, "Boy, Stop Lying and Don't Say You've Forgotten"
"The Trouble with You Is You Ain't Been Squattin"

Most meat heads, strength coaches and general fitness enthusiasts agree—squats are king!

Fortunately, the lack of a barbell is no excuse not to squat. Dumbbell squats and their variations

will blast virtually every muscle in your body.

Exercise Performance

1. Stand up straight while holding a pair of dumbbells, one in each hand facing each

   other. Set your feet approximately shoulder-width apart with your toes slightly

   pointed out.

2. Keep your head looking straight ahead.

3. With your core braced and chest up, lower your torso by pushing the hips back and

   bending the knees, maintaining an upright posture. Continue down until your thighs

   are parallel to the floor.

4. From the bottom position stand back up.

5. Repeat for prescribed number of repetitions.

Important Notes: The dumbbells can be held with a neutral grip for a hybrid squat/front squat or in the front of the body for a front squat. Dumbbell box squats, one or two-legged, are effectively utilized by many trainees.

Chapter X: Dumbbell Exercises for the Lower Leg

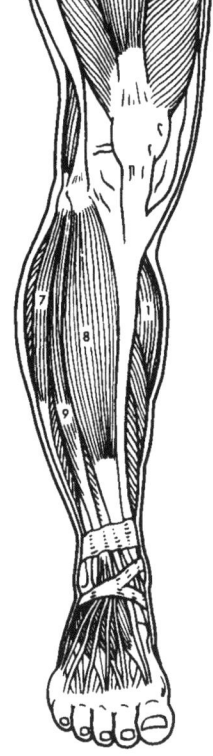 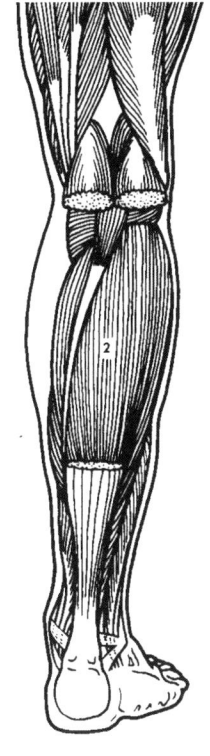 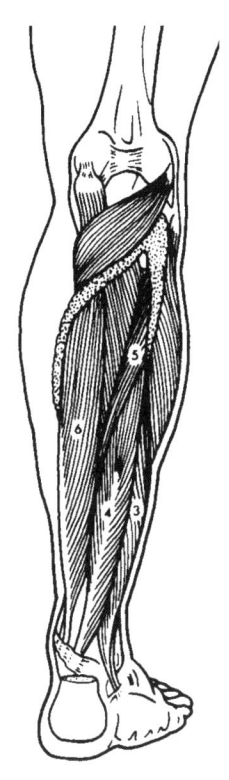

1. Gastrocnemius (Sectioned) 2. Soleus 3. Peroneus Brevis 4. Flexor Longus Hallicus 5. Tibialis Posticus	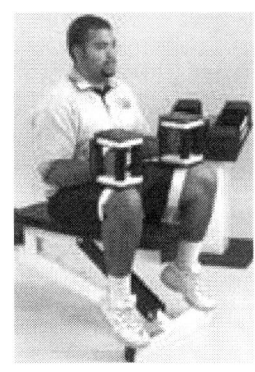	6. Flexor Longus Digitorum 7. Peroneus Longus 8. Tibialis Anticus 9. Extensor Longus Digitorum 10. Gastrocnemius (Sectioned)

In the words of the 1980s rap group Public Enemy, "Don't believe the hype!" When it comes to calf development, your genetics do not hold you prisoner. Sure, some people are blessed with great calves, but Arnold Schwarzenegger was born with the calf development of a pigeon, and through years of diligent, hard work, developed such impressive calves that he was erroneously accused of getting calf implants! This was totally false, but a great compliment.

Calf Raises

The primary action of your calf muscles (gastrocnemius) is to extend your ankle joint. However, some of the fibers also span the knee joint. In seated calf raises (shown here), those fibers are not activated. Therefore, seated calf raises are only a "good" calf exercise, and it is better to do them while your legs are not bent at the knee (i.e., while standing upright, holding the dumbbells at your side).

Standing Calf Raises

If we had to pick one calf exercise, this would be it.

Exercise Performance

1. Stand with your torso upright holding two dumbbells at your sides. Place the balls of your feet on a sturdy and stable board (approximately two to three inches) with your heels extended off and touching the floor. This is the starting position.

2. With the toes pointed straight ahead, raise the heels off the floor by contracting the calves.

3. Go back to the starting position by slowly lowering the heels.

4. Repeat for the prescribed number of repetitions.

Important Notes: To emphasize the outer head of the calves, point your toes inward and to emphasize the inner head, point your toes outward. The way to make this exercise more difficult is do it with an eccentric emphasis. This is done by performing the concentric with the same technique, but the eccentric is performed with one leg for duration of five seconds. Next perform the concentric again with two legs repeating the eccentric with one leg. Do this for the prescribed number of repetitions.

An Interesting variation:

You can also go old-school while working your gastrocs. "Donkey Calf Raises" are performed while leaning onto a high bench or table top with your training partner straddled on your hips. Like riding a donkey!

Chapter XI: Dumbbell Exercises for the Chest

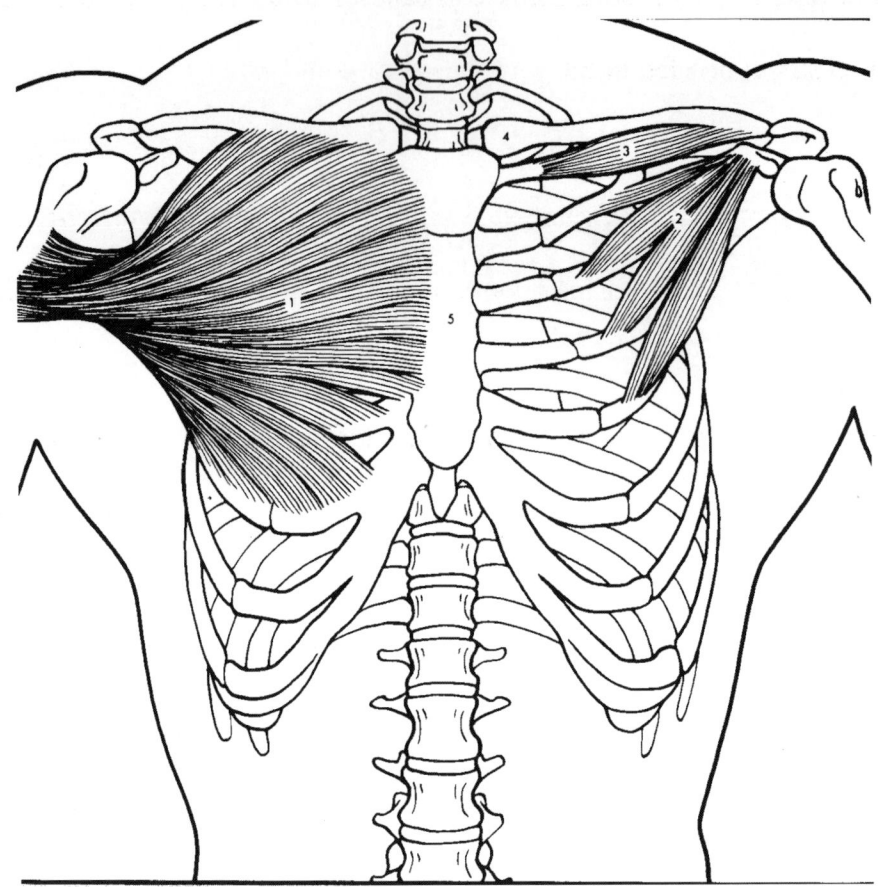

1. Pectoralis Major
2. Pectoralis Minor
3. Subclavius
4. Clavicle
5. Sternum

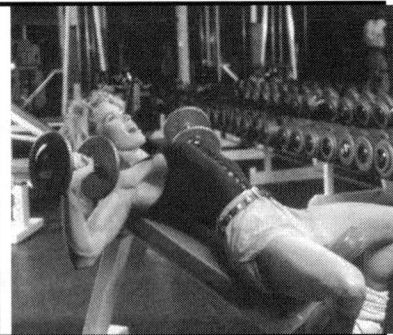

A well-developed chest is a status symbol on the prison yard weight pile or in the fancy pants

health spa.

A physique that lacks a developed chest lacks completeness and an aura of power. Many of the strongest, most powerful and muscular men of all-time have had heavy dumbbell training at the nucleus of their chest training regimens.

Dumbbell Fly

"The Austrian Oak," Arnold Schwarzenegger, largely credits the development of his chest, undoubtedly the greatest chest in the history of bodybuilding, with performance of the dumbbell fly.

The dumbbell fly is not an ego lift. The purpose of the movement is to overload the pecs through the principle of isolation. Isolation movements have fallen out of vogue with some so-called functional training experts. This is a mistake if the objective is to maximize muscular development or even create a balanced physique.

Even working and eliminating weak points can be accomplished with some isolation movements. Bottom line, faulty movement patterns are exacerbated by not eliminating weak links forcing compensatory movement patterns.

Exercise Performance

1. Lie down on a flat bench with dumbbells in each hand.

2. Lift the dumbbells above your chest with a very slight bend in the elbows, no more than 15 to 20 degrees.

3. Lower the dumbbells to your sides in an arcing motion until the chest muscles are stretched, keeping the elbows in the same fixed position. Elbow position does not change during the entire movement.

4. Bring dumbbells together in a bear hugging motion. Keep in mind, this is not a press or an extension; it is a giant hug.

5. Stop dumbbells approximately two inches short of touching.

6. Repeat prescribed repetitions.

Important notes: The stretch and technique is much more important than the weight used. Charles Poliquin advises trainees to work out with 10 percent of their bench press maximum in each hand when performing flys. This means a 400-pound bench presser would perform dumbbell flys with 40 pounds in each hand. You can shift emphasis to the upper chest region by performing flys on an incline bench. The bench should be inclined to 15 to 40 degrees. The lower portion of the chest can be attacked on a 15 to 20 degree decline bench.

Dumbbell Bench Press

For developing upper body limit strength, this movement is king! Some of the most muscular, strongest men of all time have preferred the dumbbell variation of the bench press. This elite list is not limited to, but includes: Ronnie Coleman, Branch Warren, Pat Casey and Johnnie Jackson.

Exercise Performance

1. Sitting on the end of a flat bench, with the dumbbells resting against your abdomen and thighs, carefully lie back onto the bench. Lift the dumbbells to a position directly over your chest.

2. Lower the dumbbells until they are slightly below the level of your chest and press the dumbbells to arm's length.

3. After performing the prescribed number of repetitions, lower the dumbbells back to your abdomen and sit back up so the dumbbells are again resting against your thighs and abdomen.

Important Notes: As you may have guessed, it takes a bit of practice to learn how to comfortably lie down and sit back up with the dumbbells. You will find it helpful to get assistance from a training partner until you've mastered the technique.

You can emphasize your pecs more if your elbows are away from your sides (perpendicular to your torso) during the movement. Your front deltoids are involved more if your elbows are kept close to your sides during the movement.

To further increase difficulty, you can perform this movement against resistance bands with one resistance band around your back, held in your hands along with the dumbbell. This would apply to any pressing or fly movement.

 Incline Dumbbell Bench Presses 6 kg

They are done exactly the same way as dumbbell bench presses, but with one important difference. The bench is raised from parallel to the floor to about 15 to 25 degrees. This angle allows you to target the clavicular portion of your pecs (your upper chest).

Decline Dumbbell Bench Presses X

This movement is done the same way as a dumbbell bench press, but with one difference. The bench is at a decline of 15 to 20 degrees; this angle allows you to target the sternal (or lower) portion of your chest.

Reverse Grip Dumbbell Bench Press 6 kg

For decades, the incline bench press has been the go-to exercise for building the upper chest. The lab-tested justification for this preference lies in an almost statistically irrelevant 5 percent increase in muscle activation of those upper chest fibers as compared to the flat bench press, while activity in the front delts increases by about 80 percent.

A recent Canadian study showed that the reverse grip bench press produced 30 percent more fiber activation on the upper pecs than traditional bench press.

Everything is bigger in Texas! Not surprisingly, the two most well-developed upper chests hailed from the Lone Star State: 1990s powerlifting bench press champions and record holders, Anthony Clark and Jim Voronin. Both set records with a reverse grip bench press

Exercise Performance

1. Set up for the exercise by grasping a set of dumbbells and sitting on the end of a flat bench with the dumbbells against your abdomen and thighs.

2. Lie back on the bench and place the dumbbells above your chest. Twist the dumbbells so your palms are facing your shoulders. This is your starting position.

3. Lower the dumbbells until your palms are in line with your chest, pause for half a second and press the dumbbells forcefully back up to the starting position.

4. Repeat for the specified number of repetitions.

Important Notes: Don't let the dumbbells touch at the top of each rep. Use a full range of motion at the bottom and the top of the repetition. To further shift emphasis to the upper pecs, try this movement at a 15 to 20° incline. Any routine in this book that specifies an incline press for chest development can be switched to the reverse grip bench press.

Dumbbell Pullover

The dumbbell pullover was a favorite of Arnold Schwarzenegger, Reg Park and virtually any old-timer with great chest development. Pullovers work not only the chest, but also the lats and the intercostal serratus anterior (the muscles of the rib cage). Maximally developed intercostal muscles give the illusion of a bigger rib cage when taking a deep breath and holding a pose because the ribs are pulled up by the intercostal muscles.

The elimination of pullover movements, we believe, is one of the reasons why chest development in the modern era lags behind the development of other body parts. Recent research has revealed that barbell and dumbbell pullover variations emphasize chest development, while machines more effectively target the lats.

Exercise Performance

1. Lie perpendicular to the bench press, with only your shoulders supported.

2. Your feet should be flat on the floor, shoulder-width apart. Your head and neck should hang over the bench. Your hips should ideally be at a lower angle than your shoulders.

3. Grasp a dumbbell with your hands crossed in a diamond shape with your thumbs and pointer fingers (palms should be facing the ceiling).

4. With the dumbbell over your chest and elbows bent 10 to 15 degrees (do not let this angle changed throughout the entire movement), take a deep breath, hold and slowly lower the weight backward over your head until the upper arms are in line with torso, parallel to the floor. The weight travels in an arc-like motion toward the floor.

5. Exhale and pull the dumbbell back over your chest, purposely contracting the chest muscles. Hold for a second, and repeat prescribed repetitions.

Important notes: Do this movement in a muscle-intention style, focusing on the stretch and feeling the movement. Keep reps in the 12+ range. If you have a history of shoulder problems, more than likely you will need to avoid this movement.

Chapter XII: Dumbbell Exercises for the Shoulders

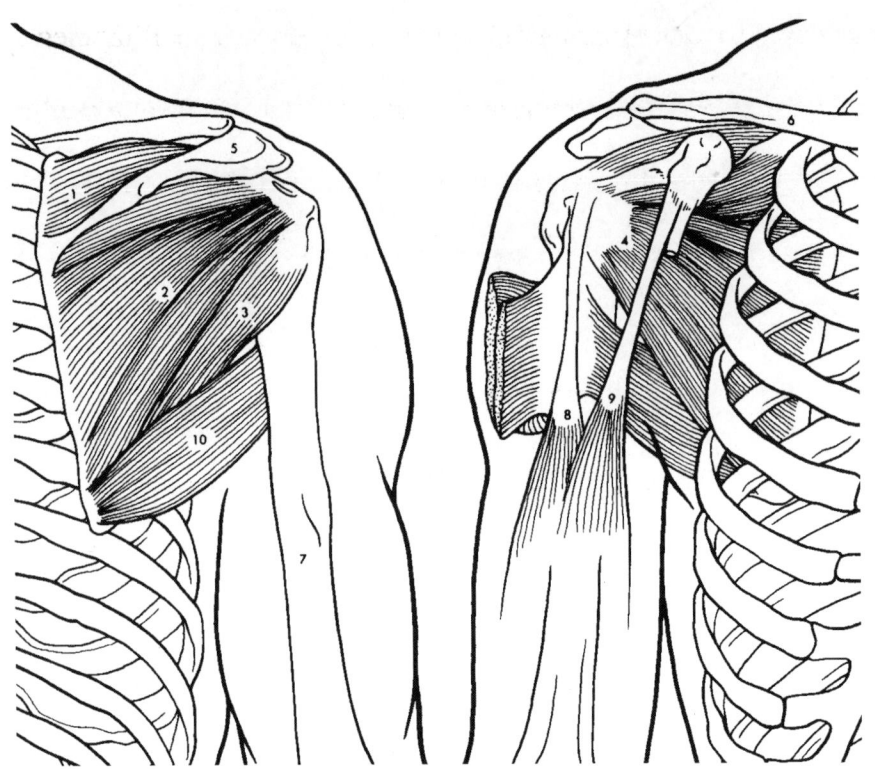

1. Supraspinatus*		6. Clavicle	
2. Infraspinatus*		7. Humerus	
3. Teres Minor*	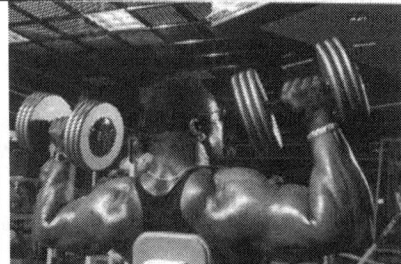	8. Biceps Brachii – Long Head	
4. Subscapularis*		9. Biceps Brachii – Short Head	
5. Spine of Scapula		10. Teres Major	

* Muscles of the Rotator Cuff

Broad, developed shoulders scream masculine virility. Wide shoulders help create the illusion of a V taper that will cause the same sex to envy you and the opposite sex to find you more attractive. Virtually every sport and recreational activity will be enhanced by increased shoulder strength and function. There is no better way to maximally develop the shoulders than with dumbbells.

Inward Rotations

Both inward and outward rotations are exercises that few incorporate into their schedule because commercial gyms rarely have the appropriate equipment. Yet rotator cuff injuries are among the most common injuries among weight trainees. Inward rotation of the rotator cuff is accomplished by the subscapularis and the teres major, with the supraspinatus acting as a stabilizer.

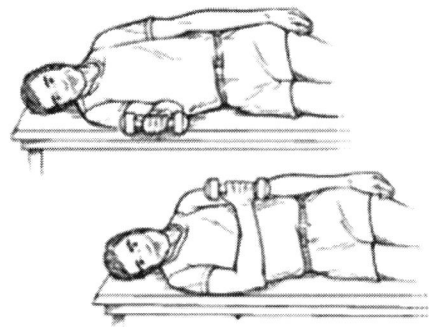

Outward Rotations

Outward rotation of the shoulder joint is accomplished by action of the infraspinatus and teres minor. As with inward rotations (described above), outward rotations are essential in preventing rotator cuff tears.

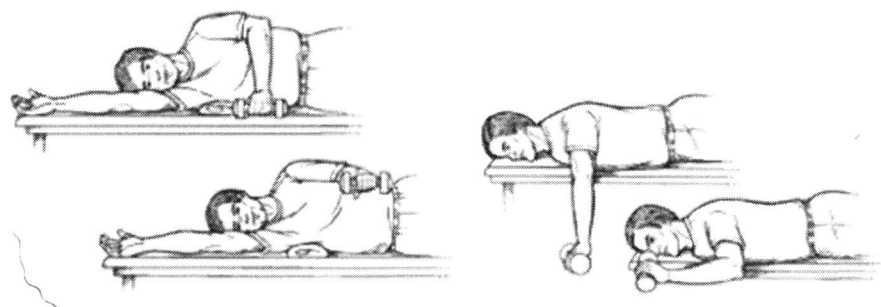

Seated Dumbbell Presses

A plethora of the strongest powerlifters and most well-developed bodybuilders consider this their bread-and-butter shoulder exercise.

Exercise Performance 4Kg   5Kg × 10

1. Grab two dumbbells and sit on a military press bench that has a back support.

2. Have a competent spotter assist you in bringing the dumbbells to shoulder height or clean the dumbbells up one at a time with the assistance of your thighs. Rotate your wrists so your palms are facing forward. This is the starting position.

3. From the starting position, push the dumbbells to full extension.

4. Lower the weight under control and repeat for the prescribed repetitions.

Important Notes: Advanced bodybuilders may opt for stopping this movement about three quarters of the way to lockout. This keeps constant tension on the deltoids without letting the triceps takeover. Other useful variations are the half, half, full. This is performed by doing two bottom half reps consecutively and on the third rep going to full extension; this sequence of three individual movements constitutes one repetition. This movement can also be performed with a neutral grip and athletes should consider performing it standing.

Arnold Press 8Kg × 10   3

The Arnold press was developed by none other than Arnold Schwarzenegger, a.k.a. "the Austrian Oak." Arnold devised this movement to help develop his medial deltoids using heavy weight.

Exercise Performance

1. Sit on a military press bench with a back support and hold two dumbbells in front of you at collarbone-level with your palms facing your body and your elbows bent (this should look similar to the top contracted position of a bicep curl).

2. Raise the dumbbells as you rotate the palms of your hands until they are facing forward (like a regular seated dumbbell military press). Continue lifting the dumbbells until your arms are extended above you.

3. From the seated position, lower the dumbbells to the original position by rotating the palms of your hands toward you.

4. Repeat for the prescribed number of repetitions.

Important Notes: Keep in mind, as the existentialists say, "Form before function."

Upright rows 2Kg 4Kg x 10

Many with Herculean shoulder development at least partially credit that development to the upright row. This movement has fallen out of favor with some in recent years and we do advise avoiding this movement if you have shoulder ailments.

Upright rows offer functional benefits to any occupation that continuously loads, like longshoreman or shelf stockers.

Exercise Performance

1. Hold two dumbbells with a shoulder-width grip. The dumbbells should be resting on top of your thighs with your arms a few degrees shy of extension.

2. Using your shoulders, lift the dumbbells to chest level with the elbows driving the motion and pause for half of a second at the top of the movement.

3. Lower the dumbbells under control to starting position.

4. Repeat for the prescribed number of repetitions.

Important Notes: Keep this exercise strict; too much weight can lead to bad form, which can lead to injury. Traditional recommendations have called for an even narrower grip than shoulder-width grip. Some new research from the University of Memphis demonstrated that a wide grip enhances the electrical activity of the medial and posterior deltoids by more than 20 percent when compared to a traditional narrow rep. Furthermore, the wider grip decreases the activity of the biceps, but increases the activity of the upper traps to maximize shoulder development.

Lateral raises

Well-developed medial (side) deltoids cap that look of complete development and power. Lateral raises have been the go-to exercise for middle deltoid development for decades. It would be very rare to find any successful bodybuilder who has not trained with lateral raises at one time or another.

Exercise Performance

1. Grab two dumbbells and stand up with your torso erect, and hold the dumbbells by your sides with your elbows slightly bent, approximately 10 to 15 degrees with your palms facing you. This is the starting position.

2. Keep the torso position stationary through the entirety of the movement. Lift the dumbbells to your side, maintaining the same elbow position throughout the entire movement.

3. Continue lifting the dumbbells with your shoulders until your arms are parallel to the floor.

4. Under control, lower the dumbbells back to the starting position.

5. Repeat for the prescribed number of repetitions.

Important Notes: One way to increase the intensity of this exercise is to perform it seated on an incline bench because of the stretch at the bottom of the movement. This provides a huge overload component, so lighter weights will have to be used. The standing variation can be effective with some slight cheating. Use just enough momentum to aid in pushing past the sticking point, but still control the eccentric. Some recent reviews in the literature have concurred with the effectiveness of cheating on standing lateral raises; do not do this on the incline variation.

Front Dumbbell Raises 14Kg 13Kg X10

Front dumbbell raises have been a favorite of Al Davis, Big Jim Williams, Bill Kazmaier, Jeremy Hoornstra and a host of some of the other greatest bench presses of all-time.

Exercise Performance

1. Hold two dumbbells resting on the front of your thighs. Your arms should have a 10 to 15-degree bend with your hands facing you (pronated grip).

2. With your right arm, lift the dumbbell in front of your body, maintaining 10 to 15 degrees of elbow flexion throughout the entire movement with your palm facing the floor; lift your arm up until the dumbbell is parallel to the floor.

3. Lower the weight, under control, to the starting position.

4. Perform front raises in an alternate fashion.

5. Repeat for the prescribed number of repetitions.

Important Notes: Some cheating, or use of momentum to get past a sticking point, is okay on this movement. Do not make it into a bastardized Olympic lift. A potentially more effective variation of this movement is to perform it with a lean before raising the dumbbell. When working your right side, lean 20 to 30 degrees to the right. Before raising the left side, lean to the left in a similar fashion. The dumbbells are raised about at arm's length in front of your face. The rationale for this departure from traditional technique is your front deltoids originate and insert at about that angle from the vertical plane of your body. Bending sideways while performing the dumbbell front raises places the targeted frontal deltoid perpendicular to the floor, thereby making its contraction (force output) more efficient. Do that and adaptive stress is increased.

Dumbbell Shrugs 6Kg

From prison politics to a sermon from the pulpit, possessing well-developed, strong traps screams power. Strong, powerful traps make one less likely to get injured in sports like rugby and football and even less likely to get knocked out trading fists at the local watering hole. Your traps elevate and support your shoulder girdle (i.e., pull the shoulders toward your ears). Shrugging builds traps by moving just straight up and down with no need for rotational movement.

Exercise Performance

1. Grab two dumbbells. Stand up straight with a dumbbell in each hand (palms facing your torso); your arms should be fully straightened.

2. Lift the dumbbells by elevating your shoulders to the highest possible position. Hold the contraction at the top position for one second. Elbows should be fully straightened through the entire movement.

3. Lower to the starting position.

4. Repeat for the prescribed number of repetitions.

Important Notes: A very effective variation of this movement is to perform it seated on a military press bench. This movement can also be performed unilaterally.

Chapter XIII: Dumbbell Exercises for the Back

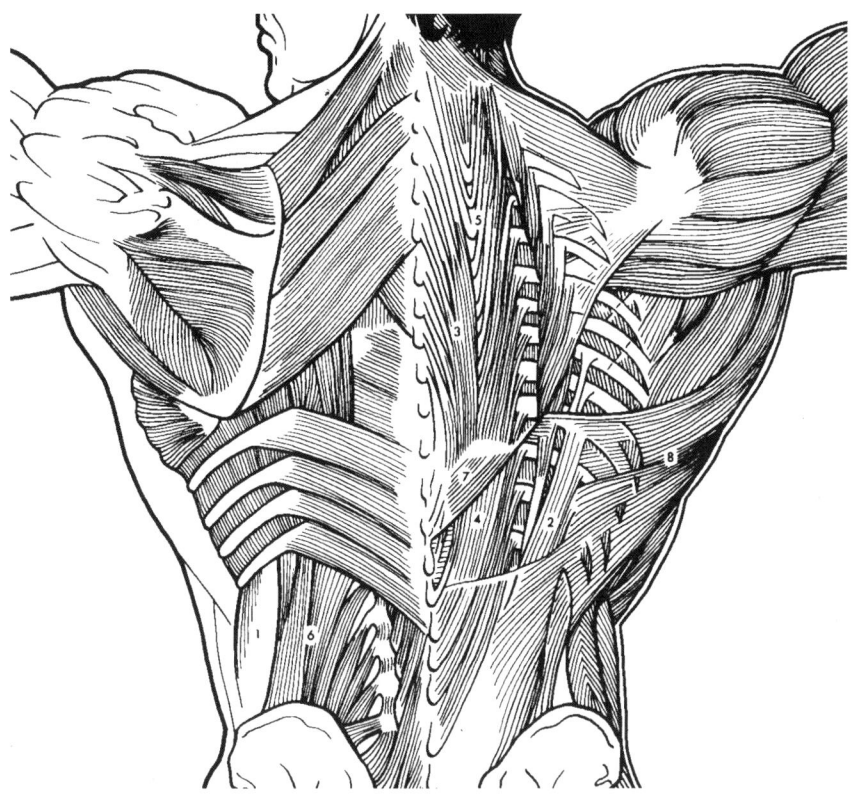

1. Internal Oblique	7. Trapezius (Sectioned)
2. Ilio-Costalis*	8. Latissimus Dorsi
3. Spinalis Dorsi*	9. Levator Anglui Scapularis
4. Longissimus Dorsi*	10. Rhomboideus Minor
5. Transversalis Cervicis*	11. Rhomboideus Major
6. Quadratus Lumborum	12. Serratus Posticus Inferior

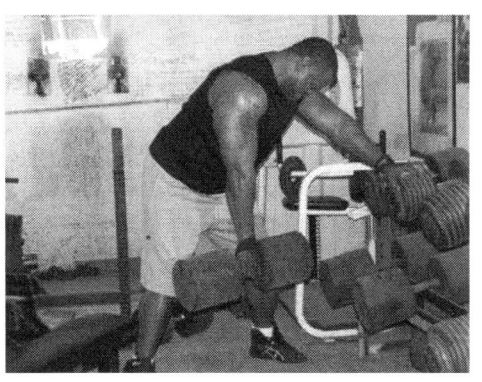

Muscles of the Erector Spinae

Ronnie Coleman, Lee Haney and Dorian Yates have the three best backs in the history of

bodybuilding, and combined, these three own nearly half of all Mr. Olympia prizes ever won.

"Strongman equals strong back," said two-time world's strongest man winner and former champion powerlifter, Bill Kazmaier.

A strong, well-developed back epitomizes functionality and projects a persona of power.

Inverted Fly 2 Kg (2½)

The inverted fly primarily targets your rhomboids. However, your posterior deltoids, trapezius III and outward rotators are also activated.

Exercise Performance

1. Grab two dumbbells with a slight bend in your knees; get in position with a flat back and your torso parallel to the floor. Dumbbells should be held palms facing (neutral grip).

2. Your arms should be nearly straight, approximately 10 degrees short of full extension. Maintain this position for the entire movement.

3. Move your arms away from each other laterally (to the side), in an arc motion, attempt to squeeze the shoulder blades together to maximize the effectiveness of the contraction, and hold the contracted position for one second.

4. Lower the weights, under control, back to the starting position.

5. Repeat for prescribed number of repetitions.

Important Notes: This exercise can also be performed face down on an incline bench press to avoid stress on the lower back. Do not make this a "cheating exercise."

One-Arm Dumbbell Rows

5 Kg + ½ Kg

This exercise has been a part of many no-nonsense power lifting and bodybuilding regimens.

Exercise Performance

1. Place a dumbbell to the side of a flat bench.

2. Place your left leg on the top of the bench; place the left hand on the other end of the bench for support. Get in position where your upper body is parallel to the floor.

3. Pick up the dumbbell with your right hand with your palm facing your torso (neutral grip). This is the starting position.

4. Using your upper back, lift the dumbbell to chest level.

5. Under control, lower the dumbbell back to the starting position.

6. Repeat for specified number of repetitions.

Important Notes: Make sure you produce the force to lift the dumbbell with your back, not your biceps or forearms. Some bodybuilders prefer this movement standing up holding on to the dumbbell rack with the non-lifting hand.

Head-Supported Dumbbell Rows 5 Kg

Head-supported rows were popularized amongst fringe bodybuilding circles by none other than the great Bill Pearl. Pearl was one of the last true bodybuilders from the era when strength mattered and performing feats of strength was an expectation, not an exception. This is one of the best movements to thicken the upper and middle back. This movement eliminates any pretense of cheating.

Exercise Performance

1. Place two dumbbells on the floor in front of your feet, which should be approximately shoulder-width apart.

2. Bend down and grab the dumbbells so that your palms are facing each other (neutral grip).

3. Place your forehead on a comfortable object that is about waist high (well-padded incline benches work well). Keep a slight bend in the legs throughout the entirety of the movement with your torso parallel to the floor.

4.	With both hands, lift the weights up using your upper back muscles. Lift the weight up as far as possible to your sides. Do not alter the position of your legs and back.

5.	Lower the weight back down to the starting position in a controlled fashion.

6.	Repeat for prescribed number of repetitions.

Important Notes: Keep your back flat and never cheat on this movement.

Dumbbell Deadlifts

This is not a popular exercise, probably because it is so dang difficult! Some powerlifters have used this movement to help build starting strength; others have used it like bodybuilders and other physique specialists to increase overload by increasing the range of motion. No matter how heavy the dumbbells are, they are much closer to the floor compared to plates on a barbell. The movement starts with a huge leverage deficit, making it much harder.

Exercise Performance

1.	Set dumbbells on the floor and stand facing the dumbbells.

2.	Bend at the hips and knees and grab the dumbbells with an overhand grip.

3.	Without allowing your back to round, stand up with the dumbbells.

4.	Lower the dumbbells back to the floor after you've achieved a fully erect position.

5.	Repeat for prescribed number of repetitions.

Important Notes: Increased ranges of motion deadlift variations were a favorite of bodybuilder Gustavo Badell, who had one of the most developed backs in pro bodybuilding in his prime. Make sure you have the mobility to perform this exercise with great technique. Do not be afraid to use wrist straps.

Weight Pull-Ups with Dip Belt and Dumbbell

This manual is about the most effective methods to train with dumbbells. However, it would not be fair not to mention you can do any pull-up or chin-up variation with a dip belt and add additional weight with dumbbells.

If you are not doing pull-ups now, start! If you are unable to do a pull-up, we recommend the book *Jailhouse Strong*, which offers a number of progression plans for the beginner to build up the strength to do pull-ups.

Chapter XIV: Dumbbell Exercises for the Upper Arms

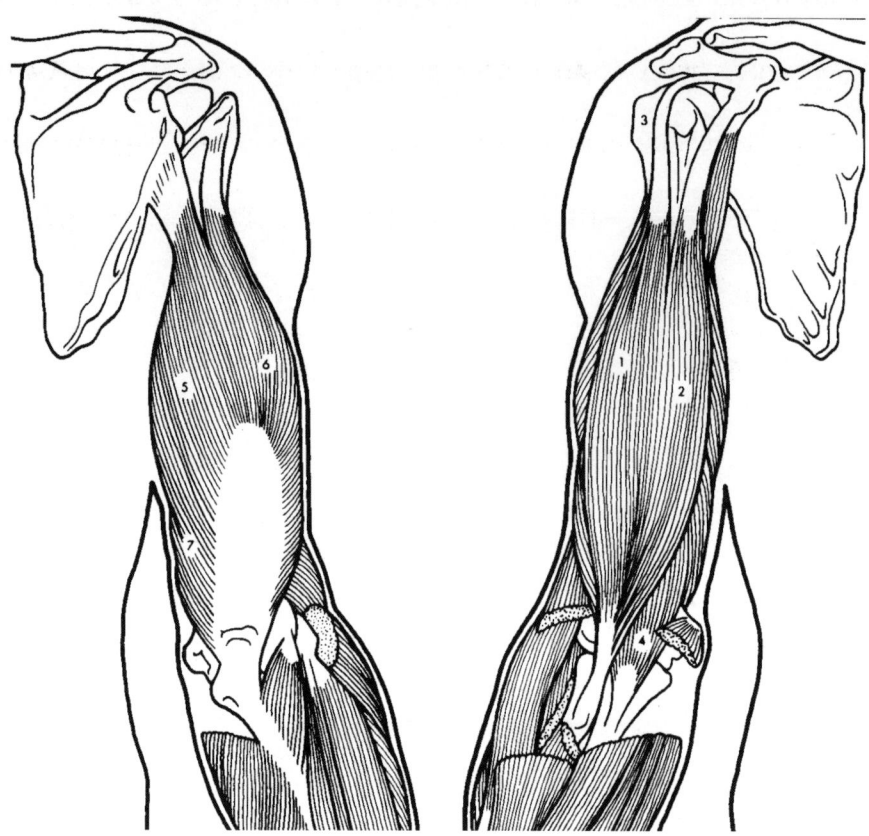

1. Biceps Brachii – Long Head 2. Biceps Brachii – Short Head 3. Head of Humerus 4. Brachialis 5. Triceps – Scapular Head 6. Triceps – Lateral Head 7. Triceps – Medial Head	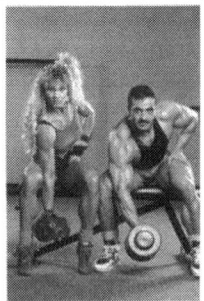

Biceps

From the immortal bodybuilding legend, Chuck Sipes, "The appreciation of big, powerful arms

is an American folk custom. By this I mean that this country was developed by the labors of all

the various pioneers and explorers over the past 300-400 years. As they pushed into the

wilderness and afterwards, wresting a living from the land, these men had to work hard, work with their hands and arms and whole body, to get along. The settler, the village blacksmith, the lumberjack, the carpenter and builder … all needed powerful arms to ply their trade well, and in time those with the greatest, most powerful arms grew to be respected for their contributions. Bodybuilding today, with the glorification of the entire well-developed physique, is still influenced by this great American heritage to the extent that big arms and powerful arms are the most respected part of the body."

This held true a half-century ago and still holds true today.

Preacher Curls

This was a favorite amongst bodybuilders in the golden era. This movement removes any sort of chance at cheating.

5 kg

Exercise Performance

1. Stand behind an incline bench.

2. Rest the back of your upper arm and elbow on the incline bench holding a dumbbell in your hand.

3. From the fully flexed position (dumbbell at shoulder level), lower the weight to the full extended position.

4. From this position, using the bicep, flex the dumbbell back to starting position.

5. Repeat for the prescribed number of repetitions.

Important Notes: Don't start from the bottom position unless you are an arm wrestler looking to develop sport-specific strength. Do not cheat the range of motion.

Zottman Curls

Zottman curls offer a terrific bang for your buck. Basically, you are performing a regular curl with an eccentric overload reverse curl, blasting the biceps and forearms into oblivion.

Exercise Performance 4Kg 5Kg×10

1. Start with one dumbbell in each hand, palms facing forward. Stand up straight with your elbows close to your torso.

2. Curl the dumbbells to your shoulders.

3. At the top of the movement, rotate your wrists with palms facing forward again. Lower the weight to the starting position using a pronated grip.

4. At the bottom, rotate your wrists again with palms facing forward.

5. Repeat for prescribed number of repetitions.

Important Note: To really blast the forearms, try this movement with Fat Gripz.

Incline Dumbbell Curls 4Kg

This movement is an extended range of motion movement. Yes, that means it's harder and no, you won't be able use as much weight with the added stretch component. This is a purposefully added overload component.

Important Notes

1. Lie back on an incline bench with the incline set at approximately 45 degrees, letting your arms hang fully extended at your sides.

2. Keep your arm supinated (palms forward) throughout the entire movement.

3. Keep your shoulders and torso stationary; curl both arms toward your shoulders as high as you can go.

4. Lower the weight to the starting position.

5. Repeat for prescribed number of repetitions.

Important Notes: Since your arms are angled behind you, the range of motion is greatly increased, adding a huge stretch component. Shortening this movement destroys the desired training effect; full range of motion for full development is the name of the game here! This exercise can be performed with both arms simultaneously or in an alternating fashion.

Hammer Curls 4Kg × 10(12)

Hammer curls have been a favorite of top powerlifters for decades. Not only to help build strong biceps, but also help strengthen the forearms to a significant degree.

Exercise Performance

1. Stand with your torso upright and a dumbbell in each hand with your arms extended, keeping the elbows close to the body.

2. Palms should be facing the torso. This is a neutral grip (that's why this grip is nicknamed Hammer grip).

3. Holding the upper arm stationary, maintaining a neutral grip, curl the weight forward contracting the biceps; continue curling to a fully contracted position. Hold the contracted position for half of a second.

4. Lower the weight, under control, to the starting position.

5. Repeat for prescribed number of repetitions.

Important Notes: This movement can also be performed seated, really focus on keeping the elbows stationary and only moving your forearms. Hammer curls can be performed bilaterally or in an alternating fashion.

Triceps

Biceps may get all the glory, but triceps are responsible for stretching the tape! Many people do not realize that the triceps account for two thirds of the upper arm, so poor triceps development is a recipe for spaghetti arms. Want to develop big, beautiful arms or press big weights? If you answered yes to one or both, you have to develop the triceps.

French Press 5Kg X10

This is an oldie but goodie! The French press exercise has been partially responsible for some of the greatest horseshoe triceps to ever grace the bodybuilding stage; it has also helped build some of the biggest "back arms on the prison tier and helped vaudevillian strongmen build huge overhead presses.

Exercise Performance

1. Standing in an erect position, grab a dumbbell overhead with both hands under the inter plate (heart-shaped grip).

2. With the elbows overhead, lower the forearms behind the head by flexing the upper arm (keep the movement at the elbow, not the shoulder).

3. Lower the weight until you feel a stretch in your triceps (top of the dumbbell should be lower than the top your head, minimally). Hold the stretched position for half of a second.

4. Extend the elbows back to starting position.

5. Repeat for prescribed number of repetitions.

Important Notes: Full range of motion is imperative on this exercise; the stretched position is part of the overload. Folks with back issues can perform this movement seated. This movement can also be performed with one arm.

Tri-set-Triceps

We were first introduced to this exercise by Joe Giandonato, MS, one of the wellness coordinators at Drexel University, who's also one of the top strength and conditioning coaches in the Philadelphia area. This movement gives new meaning to "triceps pump."

Exercise Performance

1. Grab a pair of dumbbells. Lie down on a flat bench.

2. Movement one: Perform a neutral-grip dumbbell bench press.

3. Movement two: From the top lockout position, lower your dumbbells, hinging at the elbows, to the side your head. Extend back to the lockout position.

4. Movement three: From the lockout position, lower the dumbbells behind your head (sort of like a pullover). Extend back to the starting position.

5. This three-movement sequence constitutes as one rep.

6. Repeat for prescribed number of repetitions.

Important Notes: Joe recommends starting with 35 percent of the load that you can dumbbell bench press for 10 reps (if you can do 50s, you need 17.5-pound dumbbells; in most gyms, these would not be available so you can round up to 20s or try 15s). This movement causes the extreme fatigue!

Decline Triceps Extension

Decline bench presses reduce range of motion when compared to flat bench presses. Decline triceps extensions increase range of motion. MRI studies show this movement significantly taxes all three heads of the triceps when performed with a barbell and there is no reason why the same would not hold true with dumbbells.

Exercise Performance

1. Lie on a decline bench press with two dumbbells held at arm's length extension.

2. Keeping your upper arms close to your sides and elbows stationary, bend your arms.

3. Bring the dumbbells down to the side of your head at a controlled pace until you feel a stretch in your triceps.

4. Extend the weight back up to the starting position.

5. Repeat for the prescribed number of repetitions.

Important Notes: Use a 15- to 20-degree decline and keep your elbow stationary. This is an extension, not an offshoot of a press.

Dumbbell Floor Paused Triceps Extensions

This is a great exercise to break up the eccentric/concentric chain. In other words, your triceps have to do all the work, with no help from the elastic-like energy stored on the eccentric.

Exercise Performance

1. Lie flat on the floor, holding a dumbbell in each hand. Extend your arms straight above your shoulders, palms facing each other.

2. Keep your upper arm stationary, bend your elbows and lower the weight, controlled, until the dumbbells touch the floor slightly behind your head or to the sides of your forehead.

3. Pause on the floor for one second.

4. After the pause, extend the dumbbells back to the starting position.

5. Repeat for prescribed number of repetitions.

Chapter XV: Dumbbell Exercises for the Forearms and Wrists (Grip)

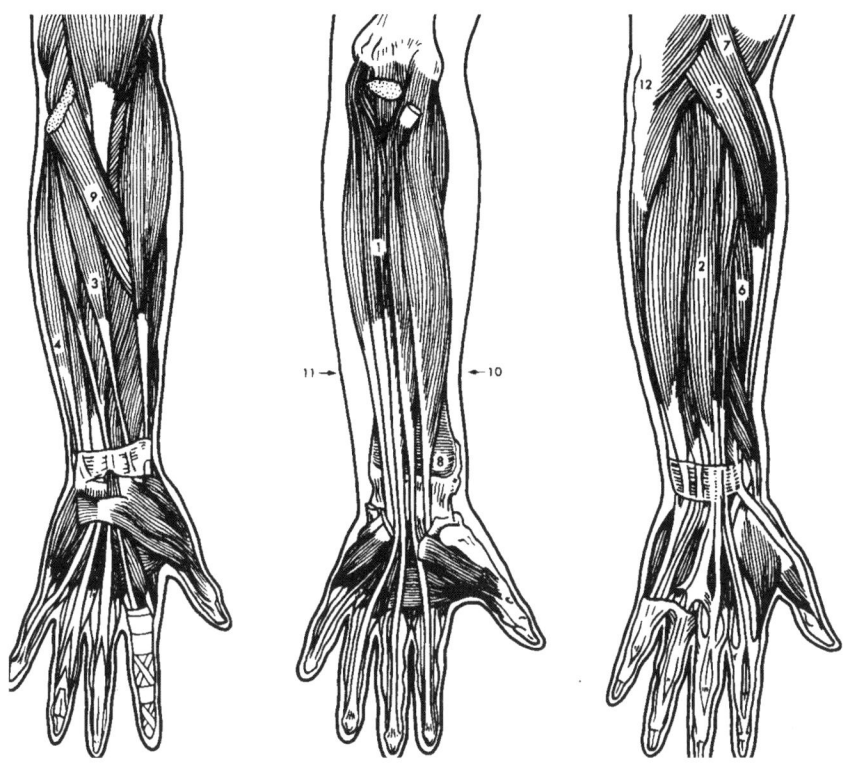

1.	Flexor Profundus Digitorum
2.	Extensor Communis Digitorum
3.	Flexor Carpi Radialis
4.	Flexor Carpi Ulnaris
5.	Extensor Carpi Radialis Longior
6.	Extensor Carpi Radialis Brevior
7.	Supinator Longus
8.	Pronator Quadratus
9.	Pronator Radii Teres
10.	Radius
11.	Ulna
12.	Elbow

A legitimately strong individual proudly wears well-developed forearms like a knight wears armor. Some of the genetically blessed get pretty good forearm development without much direct work. For the rest of us, to develop this badge of honor (big-ass forearms), we need direct work. Some of the modern day mirages of meat get their development from pumping up on chrome machines and taking scrupulous amounts of anabolic drugs. At certain poses this looks okay, but anybody who knows power, knows this façade is built by training on just machines and never having really gripped any heavy iron.

To possess the look of power, you have to have developed forearm muscles.

Wrist Curls and Reverse Wrist Curls 5Kg

A lot of sports require strong forearm muscles for grabbing, pulling, pushing or gripping. Debt collectors need these muscles to make a living, and more importantly, stay alive.

Exercise Performance

1. Sitting down, rest your right hand on your right thigh with your wrist just beyond your knees, with a dumbbell in hand (palms up/supinated grip).

2. Allow the dumbbell to roll out of your palms to your fingers, flexing at the wrist.

3. Lift the dumbbell back to the starting position by flexing the knuckles to the highest possible position.

4. Lower back down.

5. Repeat for prescribed number of repetitions (alternate sides each set).

Important Notes: This movement is very important to develop forearm flexors. Remember, the stretch is part of the movement. This is a short range of motion movement, so do not cut it shorter.

Wrist Extension

Frequently, trainees work their forearm flexors adequately, but neglect the extensors. To avoid elbow pain and not shortchange full development, it is very important to keep a balance between the extensors and flexors.

Exercise Performance

1. Sitting down, rest your right hand on your right thigh with your wrist just beyond your knees, with a dumbbell in hand (palms down/pronated grip).

2. Allow the dumbbell to roll out of your palms to your fingers, flexing at the wrist.

3. Lift the dumbbell back to the starting position by flexing up the knuckles to the highest possible position.

4. Lower back down.

5. Repeat for prescribed number of repetitions (alternate sides each set).

Important Notes: To really increase overload, try this movement with Fat Gripz.

Ulnar/Radial Deviation

A forgotten fact is that forearms do more than just extend and flex the wrist. They abduct (move away from the body) and adduct (move toward the body). For complete development, these functions must be trained.

Ulnar Deviation Exercise Technique

1. Grab a half-loaded dumbbell with the weight on the pinky side of your hand.

2. Using your wrist, move the dumbbell toward the midline of the body, moving the little finger side of the hand toward the medial side of the forearm

3. Go back to starting position.

4. Repeat for prescribed number of repetitions.

Radial Deviation Exercise Technique

1. Grab a half-loaded dumbbell with the weight on the thumb side of your hand.

2. Using your wrist, move the dumbbell laterally (away from) the midline of your body, moving the little finger side of the hand to the lateral side of the forearm.

3. Go back to starting position.

4. Repeat for prescribed number of repetitions.

Important Note: This is your ace in the hole! Ninety-nine percent of weight trainers do not work the forearms holistically.

Chapter XVI: Dumbbell Exercises for the Midsection

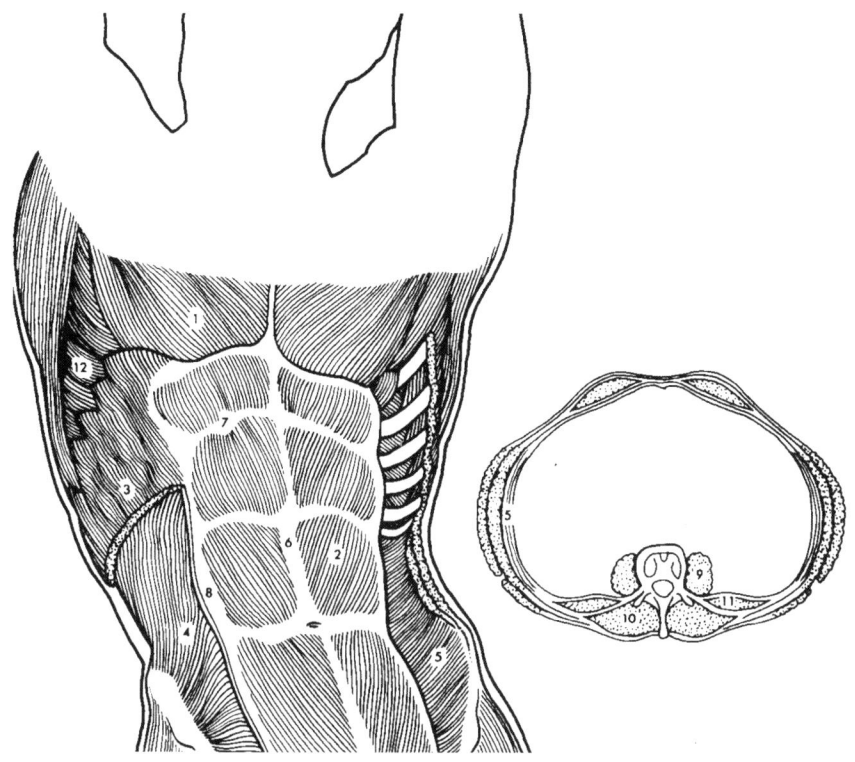

1. Pectoralis Major
2. Rectus Abdominis
3. External Obliques
4. Internal Obliques
5. Transversalis
6. Linea Alba
7. Linea Transverserae
8. Linea Similunaris
9. Psoas
10. Erector Spinae
11. Quadratus Lumborum
12. Serratus

First, stop thinking of your midsection as being comprised of just your abdominals. Of course,

that is one of the muscles of your midsection. But as the illustration above shows, there are

several other muscles that are quite important in developing a strong, shapely midsection.

Let's face it, when you're scrutinizing someone else's body—especially when much of it is exposed—your focus meanders a bit, going from here to there. However, it almost always comes back to the abs. Whether they look rock-hard or pillow-soft, they are the most obvious measure of health and fitness!

Any doubts? Compare two people whom you've never met before. One has a slovenly looking lump for a midsection, and the other has a midsection resembling corrugated steel. Now, given no additional information, who would you say is in better shape? Hell! These two people look like species from different planets! 'Nuff said.

Anatomy is Destiny

The answer to achieving that much-desired washboard appearance lies in studying the anatomy of spinal movement. This is also true of ameliorating or preventing low back pain, a condition of epidemic proportions in our culture. The particular shape any given muscle attains through the administration of progressive resistance is a result of genetic predisposition.

The spine is comprised of 33 vertebrae, only 24 of which form the flexible portion located above the sacrum. There are seven cervical vertebrae, 12 thoracic vertebrae and five lumbar vertebrae. With the exception of the first two cervical vertebrae, the extent of movement at any vertebral joint is slight, although the total movement of all joints appears to be large. The extent of movement in any given vertebral joint is due to 1) the thickness of the intervertebral discs (the larger intervertebral discs in the lumbar spine allow more movement there because they compress more), and 2) the tightness of the ligaments holding the vertebrae together (they appear to be slightly less tight in the lumbar spine).

Flexion, lateral flexion and hyperextension in the thoracic region are limited by the presence of downwardly deflected spinous processes (posteriorly) and the ribs (anteriorly). And both rotation and lateral flexion are somewhat limited in the lumbar spine because of the presence of interlocking processes. Rotation is far greater in the thoracic region.

Within these anatomical constraints, performing crunches for abdominal development involves flexion at all of the thoracic and lumbar vertebrae. Study Table One. You'll note that there are five major spinal movements possible:

- Flexion and Diagonal Flexion
- Extension and Diagonal Extension (and Hyperextension)
- Lateral Flexion
- Rotation to the Same Side
- Rotation to the Opposite Side

Table One: MOVEMENTS OF THE THORACIC AND LUMBAR SPINES

Abdominal Group	Flexion	Extension	Lateral Flexion	Rotation to the same side	Rotation to the opposite side
Rectus Abdominis	PM		Asst.		
External Oblique	PM		PM		PM
Internal Oblique	PM		PM	PM	
Psoas	Asst.*	Asst.*			
Quadratus Lumborum			PM		
Erector Spinae Group					
Iliocostalis Thoracis		PM	PM	PM	
Iliocostalis Lumborum		PM	PM	PM	
Longissimus Thoracis		PM	PM	PM	
Spinalis Thoracis		PM	PM		
Semispinalis Thoracis		PM	PM		
Deep Posterior Spinal Group					
Intertransversarii		PM	PM		
Interspinales		PM			
Rotatores		PM			PM
Multifidus		PM	PM		PM

The psoas may at times become a lumbar spine hyperextender.

In the case of the spine, rotation is always accompanied by lateral flexion, and lateral flexion is always accompanied by rotation. Circumduction (the movement of any body part that describes a "cone") is a combination of flexion, lateral flexion, hyperextension and lateral flexion to the opposite side. There is some rotation involved in spinal circumduction to the extent that it accompanies lateral flexion. All of these movements are accomplished by several muscles acting as a team, each assuming one of six possible roles:

- Prime Mover (the muscle that produces the most force to move a bone)

- Assistant Mover (the muscle that assists a prime mover in overcoming resistance)

- Antagonist (the muscle that acts in opposition to the movement occurring at the joint);

- Stabilizer (the muscle that stabilizes, or fixes, a bone so that movement can occur at another bone articulating with the stabilized bone. For example, the rectus abdominus contracts isometrically in a leg lift to stabilize the pelvis and keep it from tilting forward)

- Helping Synergist (two muscles are helping synergists when they cancel each other's normal movement, allowing the desired movement to occur)

- True Synergist (cancels the undesired movement of a prime mover while not participating in the desired movement)

Innervation for the abdominals is from the anterior divisions of the seventh, eighth, ninth, 10th and 11th dorsal nerves ("lower intercostal nerves"). They terminate in subcutaneous branches (called the anterior cutaneous nerves) near the linea alba (the abdominals' midline). The left and right sides of the rectus abdominus are separated from one another by the linea alba, and are therefore independently innervated, just as are all left and right sets of muscles of the trunk (e.g., left and right pecs).

The tendonous intersections you get after stripping away some fat and putting on some muscle are called the linea transversae. These intersections (which rarely extend across the entire abdominal wall) are located on the front of the abdominal wall only—the tendonous tissue does not separate the left or right recti into functional units. It only appears that way when viewing the "washboard" effect on an in-shape person. They are not innervated separately either, as is sometimes assumed (probably because that's the way it looks). Nor do they contract separately. Electromyographic studies have demonstrated that the upper portion of the recti produce more activity when doing crunches with no weight, but when as little as 10 pounds is added, activity is equal throughout the muscle. The same studies demonstrated that reverse crunches can produce greater activity in the lower abs than in the upper abs, but they also produce activity in the obliques. When resistance is applied to the crunch movement, differences in electrical activity disappeared and contraction became relatively uniform throughout the entire rectus abdominus. So contrary to popular belief, all abdominal exercises in which substantial resistance (weight) is being overcome will produce equally strong electromyographic activity throughout the entire muscle. In simple terms, no upper or lower part of a muscle is "isolated". In Table One, we have listed only the prime movers (PM) and assistant movers (Asst.), as these are the roles in question for developing the midsection, particularly the internal obliques, external obliques and rectus abdominus muscles.

There are many variations of abdominal exercises, and there are just as many abdominal exercise devices. All with any value, however, have one thing in common: in one way or another, they bring the ribs (origin of the abdominals) and pelvis (insertion) closer together (spinal flexion) by contracting the abdominal muscles. Your internal and external obliques aid in this movement.

These simple actions allow your abs to become a powerful "link" for your upper and lower body. With this in mind, your abs suddenly have a much more important role than simply flexing the spine or stabilizing your pelvis.

Strong abs have been well-documented to protect and support the lower back. In fact, the only longitudinal muscle responsible for maintaining a proper and healthy lumbar curvature (by stabilizing the pelvis) is your rectus abdominis. Furthermore, tight, firm abs are responsible for holding your internal organs in the proper place. This also helps support the spine.

Okay, by now you get the point. Your abs are important! The problem is, what can be done about it? Listen to 100 people, and you'll get 100 answers! Let's look at some myths that surround abdominal training.

- Myth: You can "isolate" upper and lower abs by doing crunches or reverse crunches. Not necessarily. A study done several years ago demonstrated that the upper portion of the rectus abdominis produces more activity when doing ab crunches with no weight, but when as little as 10 pounds is added, activity is equal throughout the muscle. The same study demonstrated that reverse crunches can produce greater activity in the lower abs than in the upper abs, but they also produce activity in the obliques. In simple terms, all abdominal exercises produce activity throughout the muscle; no upper or lower part of a muscle is "isolated."

- Myth: You should do high repetitions for your abs. Like all other muscles in your body, they respond best to progressive resistance training; you must train your abs like you do the rest of your muscles! And since the primary function of your abs (other than taking on the prized washboard appearance) is to stabilize your pelvis, your primary training aim should be to develop the "limit strength" of your abs. So you should use resistance. Endlessly doing reps isn't going to give you any more of a washboard appearance.

- Myth: If you use heavy weight, you'll never have a small waistline. The abdominal wall is a sheet of muscle, unlike, say, your biceps; they're not prone to bulge like a bicep is. People with large waistlines tend to have a large pelvic girdle, a beer belly, lots of fat or a combination of the three.

- Myth: Each of the abdominal segments (i.e., the washboard effect) visible on a fit individual individually flexes a different part of the spine. In a 1990s issue of a popular bodybuilding magazine, it was said that "each segment of the rectus abdominis moves or rotates a small part of the spinal column about a point known as a 'pivot point.' There are four pivot points [relating to the visible segments] along the spine. As the ab muscles contract, the pivot point moves down." This is definitely wrong! While some vertebrae flex more than others, it's a function of the anatomical structure of the spine, and *not* the result of a small portion of the abs contracting. In fact, each of the moveable vertebra in the thoracic and lumbar spine is a pivot point, and there are many more than four!

Many exercises have been developed over the ages to build abs. Some are downright harmful. Some are better than others. But as with all things in life that can be good, better or best, there is always going to be only one best way! But first, let's give due credit to all the others.

Crunches

Here's the most common crunch exercise: Lying on the floor with your legs draped over a bench, curl your head toward your knees and contract your abdominal wall so that your abs pull your ribs closer to your pelvis. Your shoulder girdle and upper back will rise up off the floor in the process. Don't raise your lower back up off the floor. Use a weight plate behind your head or resting on your upper chest if this movement is too easy for you.

There are many crunch machines on the market nowadays that simulate the crunch technique described above. The better-known ones are listed in the table below. Most are "good." The best ones, however, add a feature to the exercise that was first seen during the early 1970s (in the first generation Nautilus machines) and again a few years ago (Scorpion Equipment)—a head-support feature.

Why support the head? Well, since most heads weight 14 to 16 pounds (more or less), it can be pretty stressful on the muscles and cervical vertebrae supporting that ponderous globe! The sternocleidomastoid, assisted by the three scaleni muscles and the prevertebral muscle group (longus coli, longus capitis, rectus capitis anterior and rectus capitis lateralis), is responsible for cervical flexion—bringing the head forward (or up if you're lying down on your back). Among detrained individuals, this action can cause neck strain resulting in vertebral subluxation.

Reverse Crunches

This exercise has the same basic effect as crunches. However, your knees come toward your face instead of vice versa. Some bodybuilders believe that they can get better lower abdominal development with this exercise. We personally doubt it because the research tends to refute this age-old myth. So does empirical observation. Ever see a guy with great washboard upper abs but a saggy lower abdomen? Or vice versa? No such thing! It's more tenable that the entire abdominal wall benefits equally from either exercise.

You can make this exercise more difficult by raising the incline board that you're lying on a bit higher. Begin with your knees and hips completely flexed. When raising your knees toward your face, you shouldn't swing them upward, as the ballistic movement will tend to remove some of the desired stress. Instead, raise them up.

Russian Twists

During the Soviet era, the Russians were famous for their great athletes. One of the exercises that all Russian athletes do for the abdominal muscles, the internal oblique muscles and the external oblique muscles has become known as the Russian Twists. Every time you twist, swing a bat, or throw, you use these important muscles. As for its usefulness to bodybuilders, this exercise tightens the entire midsection in a girdle effect. Your obliques will probably never grow so large that they bulge out (called "Apollo's Girdle"). But it's possible, provided your genetics predispose such massive growth potential.

Your lower back remains in contact with the ground (or, better yet, in contact with an "S.I. pad" tucked under your sacroiliac, or lower back), and your feet are positioned close to your buttocks (knees bent). Holding a small weight directly over your face at arms' length, twist all the way to the right and then to the left several times. Do not allow your torso or shoulders to come in contact with the ground while twisting left and right. And don't deviate laterally from your longitudinal axis.

Hanging Leg Raises

The myth is that hanging while raising your knees upward is going to selectively develop your lower abs. Actually, hanging leg raises are the ultimate version (the highest stress version) of reverse crunches. Reread the description of reverse crunches, and then attempt to do hanging leg raises. Bet you can't! The only people we've ever seen capable of doing this exercise correctly are accomplished gymnasts.

Your best bet is to do reverse crunches. Remember, flexing your hips during the knee raise is developing your hip flexors (iliopsoas) and your grip (forearm) muscles, not your abs!

Sidebends

Here's yet another preventive exercise for your spine! This time, you're exercising two very large muscle groups that help stabilize your lower back—your obliques and your quadratus lumborum muscles. Both are extremely important to bodybuilders and athletes alike in that they must be strong to prevent back injuries.

Of course, bodybuilders benefit from the fact that (as with Russian Twists) the "Apollo's Girdle" effect comes into play. Your toned obliques will tend to "trim" your waist. Simply bend directly sideward toward the side holding the dumbbell. The other arm is behind your head to pre-stretch your targeted obliques.

Some of these exercises are good, meaning they're better than doing nothing. Some of these exercises are really good. But I've saved the best for last. All of the aforementioned exercises involve partial movements or movement where the rectus abdominus, internal obliques or external obliques contract in a static state. These conditions do not produce the "best" results.

Partial Movements vs. Full Range Movements

Partial movements have their place in weight training. Bodybuilders use them when working on limit strength or sticking points, and athletes in many sports use them for both these purposes as well as in simulating sports-specific movements. However, it's safe to say that full-range movements are generally more productive in improving strength, tone and mass. So let's explore one of the reasons why full-range movements are so productive. It has to do with the amount of work being accomplished.

Let's say you squat with 500 pounds, but only go half way down. Your normal "stroke" (distance over which you move the weight) equals two feet, but you only go one foot down. And, let's say the upward movement takes one second.

Power = force × distance ÷ time

P = 500 × 1 foot ÷ 1 second = 500

Now, let's say you did the full squat movement of two feet in the same amount of time:

P = 500 × 2 feet ÷ 1 second = 1000.

Clearly, you've done twice the amount of work:

Work = force × distance

Work = 500 × 2 = 1000

Even if it took you twice the amount of time to perform the full range of movement, you've still done twice the work:

P = 500 × 2 feet ÷ 2 seconds = 500, but

Work = 500 × 2 feet = 1000.

You don't have to be a rocket scientist to understand that twice the work makes for a much more efficient workout! But, let's look at one more reason why full-range movements are often more productive in bodybuilding and sports. This time, we'll look at what's going on at the cellular level—inside the contracting muscle itself.

When you stretch a muscle to its full length, the myofibrillar elements (actin and myosin) are fully stretched. That means that the overlap between the actin and myosin myofibrils is minimal, and you're not as capable of producing force. Remember, the cross-bridging going on between the actin and myosin strands is what causes contraction.

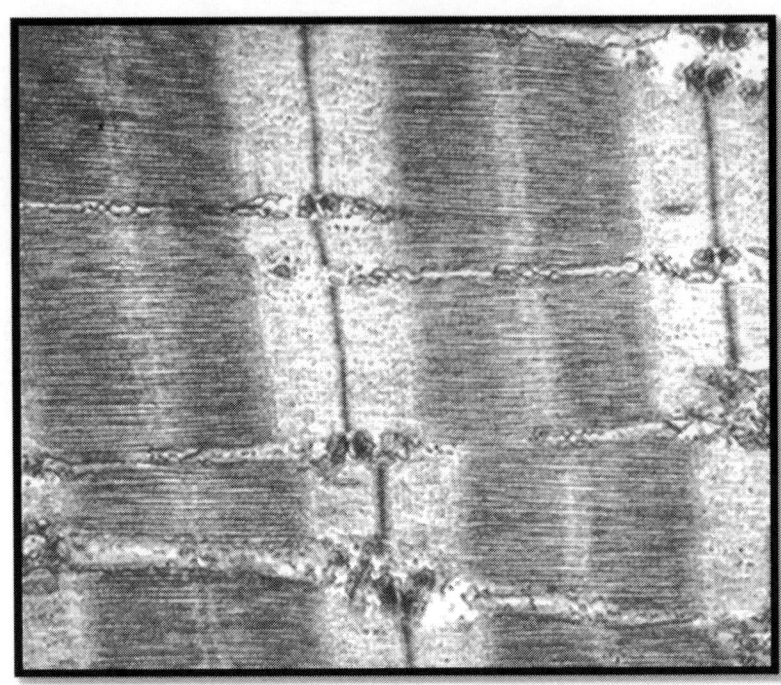

The light and dark stripes are a result of the greater or lesser overlap of these myofibrils. Thus, a fully contracted muscle would appear darker than a muscle that was fully stretched.

Over a few weeks of time, however, the actin and myosin myofibrils adapt to this new requirement of having to produce force while stretched. They do so by growing longer in an attempt to increase the amount of overlap between them. This, of course, has the net effect of increasing the amount of force you can generate even while stretched!

The photo below of a spine being manipulated illustrates the amount of flexion each of the vertebrae is capable of. You can see that there is a two- to three-degree movement capability between each thoracic vertebral joint and three to five degrees of movement possible between each lumbar vertebral joint. It's clear that a full range crunch movement from about 30 degrees hyperextension to about 30 degrees hyperflexion is quite possible. You can accomplish this by placing a few rolled up towels behind your lumbar spine while doing full range crunches.

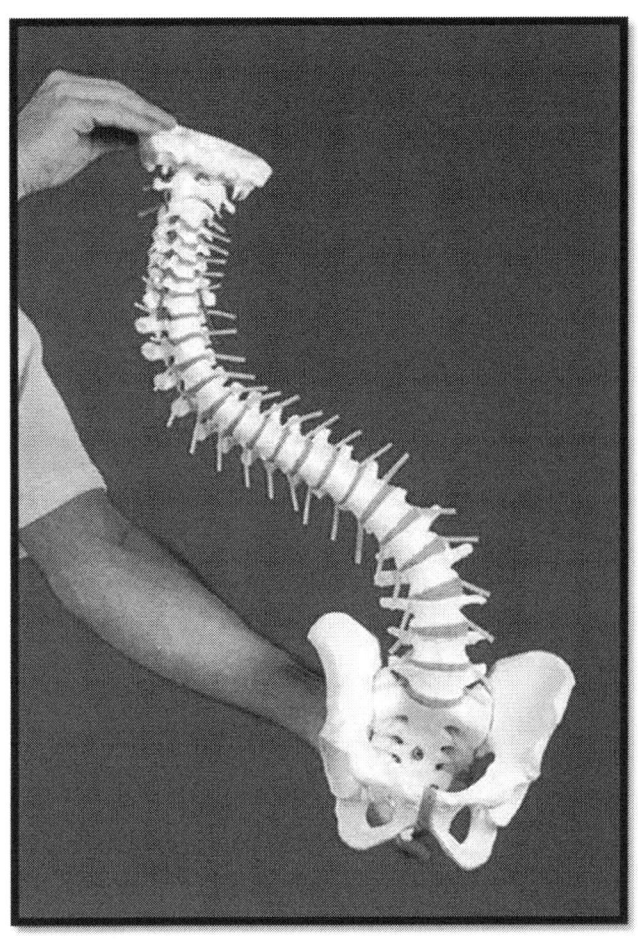

Of course, another is that the amount of work you're accomplishing is virtually doubled. Your

thoracic vertebral joints are capable of a few degrees of flexion and hyperextension, and the

lumbar vertebrae slightly more. The curvature of your padded "bench" closely matches the range

of movement intended for your thoracic and lumbar spines. This ensures non-traumatic

movement from an unforced hyperextended position to an unforced flexed position. And this

ensures the greatest possible range of motion and the least possible intervertebral trauma.

For those of you with bad backs (almost all of you, if statistics can be trusted), it has become

axiomatic that ab work is the best therapy for your condition. And for those of you whose backs

are virgin to troublesome herniations, subluxations and ruptures, it is as much the case for

prevention.

A few points to ponder:

- You can't put your obese client on the ground to do crunches without causing severe psychological trauma (it's embarrassing to them when they try to get up or down).

- The ab machines on the market are difficult to get into and out of, are principally hip flexors (the abs are forced to statically contract while the iliopsoas contracts to bring your torso forward or your knees toward your chest), and –they involve only a half range movement capability.

- Full-range crunches are 100 percent more productive than half range crunches.

- Decompression of the intervertebral discs during the pre-stretched crunch movement is desirable.

- Abdominal muscle cells are no different from other muscle cells, and therefore will respond optimally based on the specific fiber type(s) comprising the muscle.

- Prestretched ab crunches are the only exercise capable of solving all these problems.

- Don't neglect the critical importance of diet and nutrition! The only way you (or anyone else) will ever get to see your six-pack is if you strip the ugly fat away! That means careful dieting!

- Now for the big question: What to do with those sensitive obese clients? Have them do their crunches on an incline bench! Adjust it up or down, depending on their ability, and fashion a pad (a rolled up beach towel, for example) for their low back so that they can get some hyperextension (to increase their range of motion during exercise). Voila!

Chapter XVII: Training Programs

ABC System of Periodized Bodybuilding

The ABC system of bodybuilding training is a program based on the Seven Granddaddy Laws of training. These rules are not new, nor can anyone claim to have discovered them. Over the years, these rules have gained acceptance as "laws"; they are set in stone.

While Dr. Hatfield and the International Sports Sciences Association have noted them, every other credible expert in the training sciences acknowledges them, even if they have different names for them.

THE ABC SYSTEM IS NOT SET IN STONE—THE PRINCIPLES BEHIND IT ARE!

For example, we will present programs that are meant to be applied three days per week and five days per week and ABC approaches that focus on movements rather than body parts.

The program outlined below is definitely doable, even for folks with busy lives. Sure, you will need dedication and you may have to train in the evening or early in the morning to fit it in. It is seven days a week and we don't feel sorry for you! As we said, we will give you alternatives that follow the universally accepted rules of training. But 99 percent of the population can, if they are dedicated, follow this program. None of the workouts in this program should be longer than 90 minutes. Most of them are 20 to 35 minutes long, unless you are exercising your jaw muscles too much between sets!

Tables 1 and 2 give you a 28-day schedule. Following that are the workouts to be done on each day.

Table 1.

Exercise	Day													
	1	2	3	4	5	6	7	8	9	10	11	12	13	14
Legs	A				B					C				
Chest		A			B				C					B
Shoulders		B			A		B			C				B
Triceps		C				B			A		B			C
Back	C					B				A				B
Biceps			A		B			C				B		
Forearms	A		A		A		A		A		A		A	
Calves	A		A		A		A		A		A		A	
Abs		A		A		A		A		A		A		A

Table 2.

Exercise	Day													
	15	16	17	18	19	20	21	22	23	24	25	26	27	28
Legs		B					A				B			
Chest				A			B				C			
Shoulders			A		B			C				B		
Triceps				A		B			C				B	
Back				A			B				C			
Biceps	A	B				C				B			C	
Forearms		A		A		A		A		A		A		A
Calves	A		A		A		A		A		A		A	
Abs		A		A		A		A		A		A		A

Legs

For this body part, our staple exercise will be the Keystone Deadlift. With that in mind, you can break the legs down into hamstrings, quadriceps, glutes and lower back, in the same fashion we did with the upper body (chest, shoulders and triceps, with the main exercise the bench press). If you decide to do so, give the same amount of rest time to each muscle as listed in the chart for legs.

Examples

A. **Workout**—Keystone Dumbbell Deadlifts 65 percent/6 reps × 3 sets

B. **Workout**—Keystone Dumbbell Deadlifts 75 percent × 6 × 3, Sissy Squats 8 × 2

C. **Workout**—2 giant sets: Keystone Dumbbell Deadlift 80 percent × 5, Dumbbell Lunges 65 percent 12, Free Squats BW × 40

Chest

We understand it's as tough to isolate the pecs from the shoulders and triceps as it is to isolate the various leg muscles. We will do our best, but realize it will still cut into recovery time of the other muscles. In the general notes section, we point out that you can move workouts around so that they work in harmony.

It may be advantageous to use a wider grip (elbows out) on the bench press so that the pectorals get the brunt and not the shoulders or triceps. You could even use exercises like the pec deck or dumbbell flys instead.

Examples

A. **Workout**—Dumbbell Bench Press 65 percent/6 × 3

B. **Workout**—Dumbbell Bench Press 75 percent/6 × 3,Chest Flys 65 percent/12 × 2

C. **Workout**—2 giant sets: Dumbbell Bench Press 80 percent × 5, Chest Flys 65 percent × 12, Dumbbell Reverse Grip Bench 35 percent × 40

Shoulders

Shoulders, like triceps, must coincide with the chest exercises if we are using the bench press as our main chest exercise. Moving exercises a day ahead or a day later is not that big of a deal.

If you are benching with a wide grip, you should still be able to fit these exercises in on their prescribed days. If you don't feel comfortable with that, then by all means move them to another day.

Examples

   A. **Workout**—Front Raises 6 × 3
   B. **Workout**—Front Raises 6 × 3, Lateral Raises 12 × 2
   C. **Workout**—2 giant sets: Front Raises × 6, Lateral Raises × 12, Dumbbell Overhead Press × 40

Triceps

The commentary provided in the chest and shoulder section also applies to tricep work. Here are the workouts:

Examples

   A. **Workout**—Decline Dumbbell Triceps Extension 12 × 3
   B. **Workout**—Decline Dumbbell Triceps Extension 12 × 2, Bar Dips 6 × 2
   C. **Workout**—2 giant sets: Bar Dips × 6, Decline Dumbbell Triceps Extension × 6, Tate Press × 40

Back

There are two approaches you can take in training the back. You can use bent rows and work the posterior deltoids and rhomboids, or you can work the lats. Of course, you could do them both! Like the bench press, your biceps will also be trained with some of the movements. Keep that in mind and make adjustments as needed.

Examples

   A. **Workout**—Dumbbell Bent Row 6 × 3
   B. **Workout**—Pull-ups 6 × 3, Dumbbell Bent Row 6 × 3, Seated Dumbbell Shrugs 12 × 2

> C. **Workout**—2 giant sets: Pull-ups × 12, Dumbbell Bent Row × 6, Reverse Fly × 12, Pull over × 40, Seated Dumbbell Shrugs 12 × 2

Biceps

On the 40 × 2 sets, use dumbbells with both arms working together at the same time to ensure constant tension, which is a must for what you want to achieve by doing them.

Examples

A. **Workout**—Dumbbell Curls 6 × 3

B. **Workout**—Dumbbell Curls 6 × 3, Zottman Curls12 × 2

C. **Workout**—2 giant sets Dumbbell Curls × 6, Zottman Curls × 12, Incline Dumbbell Curls × 40

Forearms, Calves, Abs

These muscles are predominately slow-twitch and therefore can be trained often, so you can work them in the ABC approach or in staggered sets throughout the week, i.e., when it's best for you.

Guidelines

You may find it advantageous to move a workout up a day or back a day. A general rule of thumb is to move workouts that work larger muscles like the pectorals back and workouts using smaller muscles like the shoulders or triceps up a day.

1. This system is very intense! Proper sleep, nutrition and supplementation are a must.

2. Listen to your body. You may find that you don't need as much recovery as we suggested or you may need an extra day. Listening to your body is a good thing—just don't let it lie to you! Laziness is not a reason!

3. A giant set (C workouts) is a set of five reps, a set of 15 reps and a set of 40 reps done without rest between sets. Furthermore, there is no rest between giant sets. This means you will be doing 130 reps in a row with no rest. Of course, you can take time to change

weights and move to a different exercise, but that is a matter of 5 to 10 seconds. Yes, it can be done! You may need to lower the weight used a bit, but not much.

4. The 40 reps in a giant set are slow (2/2 cadence, but that is not a strict rule) and continuous. Don't stop between reps! A slight pause between the other sets is okay.

5. Realize we are presenting merely guidelines, so the percentages are not contradictory to what was discussed earlier; they are averages. An A day is slight stimulation, B day is strong stimulation and a C day is annihilation. Adjust as needed.

Others may not want to train daily. Here is an ABC training guide for three days a week. Remember, as with the other programs, this one is not set in stone, only the concept of periods of high intensity followed by periods of low intensity, as well as the other six rules of training. Tables 1 and 2 outline an eight-week program using a three-day per week training routine.

Table 1.

Body Part	Week 1			Week 2			Week 3			Week 4		
	M	W	F	M	W	F	M	W	F	M	W	F
Legs	A	A	B	C		B	A	A	B	C		B
Chest	C		B	A	A	B	C		B	A	A	B
Shoulders		A	B	C		B	A	A	B	C		B
Back	C		C	A	A	B	C		B	A	A	C
Arms	A	C		A	C		A	C		A	C	
Abs	A	A	A	A	A	A	A	A	A	A	A	A
Calves	A	A	A	A	A	A	A	A	A	A	A	A

Table 2.

Body Part	Week 5			Week 6			Week 7			Week 8		
	M	W	F	M	W	F	M	W	F	M	W	F
Legs	A	A	B	C		B	A	A	B	C		B
Chest	C		B	A	A	B	C		B	A	A	B
Shoulders		A	B	C		B	A	A	B	C		B
Back		A	B	A	A	B	C		B	A	A	B
Arms	C		B	A	A	B	A	C			A	B
Abs	A	A	A	A	A	A	A	A	A	A	A	A
Calves	A	A	A	A	A	A	A	A	A	A	A	A

Pros and Cons

The pro of this format is it can be easier to fit into a rigid schedule. A big complaint of many trainees with the ABC approach is they claim they can't get into the gym every day. This format is much easier to put into a regular and busy weekly work schedule; this is easier to schedule around life's events.

The con of this format is that it isn't as productive as if you have a more flexible schedule. Not all muscles recover at the same rate, yet if you are going to stick to a set schedule; you may be forced to wait a day before training when you may not need it. For example, you may need four full days to recover from your C leg workout, but perhaps only three full days are needed for arms. That is not optimal training, but it can be a fair tradeoff to have a fixed schedule of training.

With this training program, you should make adjustments as you see fit. Listen to what your body is telling you, unless you have a track record of being lazy! Nothing is set in stone as long as the Seven Training Principles aren't violated.

Can ABC training be used in a format that only uses two workouts per week? Sure! Monday could be an A or B workout and Thursday could be a C workout. It'll work, but remember: Strength and size come with training frequently. For maximum results, you must train as hard and as often your ability to recover will allow. You can't always train hard, which is one of the major reasons for using an ABC approach. Regardless, training for maximum results often means getting enough rest, eating properly and supplementing your diet.

Some of the high-intensity techniques talked about earlier for advanced bodybuilders can most certainly be integrated into the ABC program; these would have to be integrated into a C day.

Seven Granddaddy Law Review

In case you are not familiar with the Seven Granddaddy Laws of training, or need a review, here is a short recap.

1. **The Law of Individual Differences**: We all have different abilities, bodies and weaknesses, and we all respond differently (to a degree) to any given system of training. These differences should be taken into consideration when designing your training program.

2. **The Overcompensation Principle:** Mother Nature overcompensates for training stress by giving you bigger and stronger muscles.

3. **The Overload Principle:** To make Mother Nature overcompensate, you must stress your muscles beyond what they're already used to.

4. **The SAID Principle:** Specific Adaptation to Imposed Demands—Each organ and organelle responds to a different form of stress.

5. **The Use/Disuse Principle:** "Use it or lose it" means that your muscles hypertrophy with use and atrophy with disuse.

6. **The GAS Principle:** The acronym for General Adaptation Syndrome, this law states that there must be a period of low-intensity training or complete rest following periods of high-intensity training.

7. **The Specificity Principle:** You'll get stronger at squats by doing squats as opposed to leg presses, and you'll get greater endurance for the marathon by running long distances than you will by say cycling long distances.

Sample Workouts Using Dumbbells

In the example program below, you will see relatively common exercises that are routinely performed nowadays by gym folk everywhere. As a testament to the fact that the science of dumbbell training has advanced considerably since the early 1900s, *none* of the exercises below was included in Professor Barker's amazing course!

An Example of a Dumbbell Training Program (6 Days per Week)

Monday (Chest, Shoulders, Upper Back)

- Dumbbell Bench Presses (Chest)

- Lateral Dumbbell Raises (Middle Delts)

- One Arm Dumbbell Rows (Posterior Delts, Lats)

- Dumbbell Shrugs (Traps)

Tuesday (Legs, Arms, Midsection)

- Front Lunge Walking with Dumbbells (Quads, Gluteals)

- Keystone Deadlifts with Dumbbells (Hamstrings)

- Dumbbell Toe Raises (Claves)

- Dumbbell Curls (Biceps)

- French Presses with Dumbbells (Triceps)

- Forward and Reverse Wrist Curls (Forearms)

- Dumbbell Side Bends Left and Right (Internal and External Obliques)

- Crunches (Abdominals)

Wednesday (Chest, Shoulders, Upper Back)

- Dumbbell Flys (Chest)

- Front Dumbbell Raises (Anterior Delts)

- Inverted Dumbbell Flys (Rhomboids)

Thursday (Legs, Arms, Midsection)

- Side Squats with Dumbbells (Quads, Gluteals, Adductors)

- Dumbbell Stiff-Legged Deadlifts (Hamstrings, Spinal Erectors)

- Dumbbell Toe Raises (Claves)

- Dumbbell Hammer Curls (Biceps, Brachialis)

- Dumbbell Dips (Triceps)

- Forward and Reverse Wrist Curls (Forearms)

- Crunches (Abdominals)

Friday (Chest, Shoulders, Upper Back)

- Dumbbell Bench Presses (Chest)

- Lateral Dumbbell Raises (Middle Delts)

- One-Arm Dumbbell Rows (Posterior Delts, Lats)

- Dumbbell Shrugs (Traps)

Saturday (Legs, Arms, Midsection)

- Front Lunge Walking with Dumbbells (Quads, Gluteals, Hamstrings)

- Keystone Deadlifts with Dumbbells (Hamstrings)

- Dumbbell Toe Raises (Claves)

- Dumbbell Curls (Biceps)

- French Presses with Dumbbells (Triceps)

- Forward and Reverse Wrist Curls (Forearms)

- Dumbbell Side Bends Left and Right (Internal and External Obliques)

- Crunches (Abdominals)

Variable Split System

Note: while it's okay to work the lower back on the same day as legs, you should never do lower back workout the day before or the day following leg workouts.

Note: while it's okay to work biceps on the same day as upper back, you should never do biceps the day before or the day following upper back workouts.

VARIABLE SPLIT SYSTEM

Including days of recovery required for each body part before training it again,
and the recommended exercises for each body part

Body Part	"Easy" Workouts	"Moderate" Workouts	"Heavy" Workouts
Chest	2 Days Rest After Incline Bench Press	3 Days Rest After Dumbbell Bench Press	4 Days Rest After Dumbbell Bench Press Incline Bench Press
Shoulders	2 Days Rest After Seated Dumbbell Presses	3 Days Rest After Front Dumbbell Raises Seated Dumbbell Presses	4 Days Rest After Front Dumbbell Raises Seated Dumbbell Presses Inverted Flyes
Traps		3 Or 4 Days Rest Dumbbell Shrugs	
Lower Back	3 Days Rest After Dumbbell Back Raises	4 Days Rest After Dumbbell Back Raises Stiff-Legged Deadlifts	5 Days Rest After Dumbbell Back Raises Stiff-Legged Deadlifts Sidebends Left and Right
	(Note: while it's okay to work the lower back on the same day as legs, you should never do lower back workout the day before or the day following leg workouts)		
Upper Back	2 Days Rest After Bent Rows (Elbows Out) Bent Rows (Elbows In)	3 Days Rest After Bent Rows (elbows Out) Bent Rows (Elbows In)	4 Days Rest After Bent Rows (Elbows Out) Bent Rows (Elbows In) Inverted Flyes
Biceps	2 Days Rest After Dumbbell Preacher Curls	3 Days Rest After Seated Incline Dumbbell Curls	4 Days Rest After Dumbbell Curls
	(Note: while it's okay to work biceps on the same day as upper back, you should never do biceps the day before or the day following upper back workouts)		
Triceps	2 Days Rest After Kickbacks	3 Days Rest After Kickbacks French Presses	4 Days Rest After Kickbacks French Presses
	(Note: while it's okay to work triceps on the same day as chest, you should never do triceps the day before or the day following chest workouts)		
Midsection	2 Or 3 Days Rest After Weighted Pre-stretched Crunches Russian Twists		
Quadriceps & Hamstrings	3 Days Rest After Walking Lunge Squats	4 Days Rest After Walking Lunge Squats One Legged Side Squats	5 Days Rest After Dumbbell Step-Ups One Legged Side Squats Keystone Deadlifts
	(Note: quad and ham workouts typically best if done together)		
Calves	2 Or 3 Days Rest Seated Calf Raises or Standing Calf Raises		
Forearms	2 Or 3 Days Rest Wrist Curls (Flexions) Reverse Wrist Curls (Extensions)		

Final Thoughts

We really appreciate the opportunity to be a part of your fitness-training process. You have been given the tools to be able "to fish." If your appetite is to eat today and you're ready to go to the gym, you have been provided the blueprint. These techniques we have presented have been used by world-class athletes under our tutelage for decades. We believe in providing you, the reader, with the best. Good luck with your journey! Time to hit the pig iron!

Printed in Great Britain
by Amazon